Kidney Disease

Heal Your Kidneys & Reverse Kidney Disease Naturally

(Ten Most Important Things Everyone Must Know About Their Kidneys)

Brain Hayes

Published By **Elena Holly**

Brain Hayes

All Rights Reserved

Kidney Disease: Heal Your Kidneys & Reverse Kidney Disease Naturally (Ten Most Important Things Everyone Must Know About Their Kidneys)

ISBN 978-1-77485-547-8

No part of this guidebook shall be reproduced in any form without permission in writing from the publisher except in the case of brief quotations embodied in critical articles or reviews.

Legal & Disclaimer

The information contained in this ebook is not designed to replace or take the place of any form of medicine or professional medical advice. The information in this ebook has been provided for educational & entertainment purposes only.

The information contained in this book has been compiled from sources deemed reliable, and it is accurate to the best of the Author's knowledge; however, the Author cannot guarantee its accuracy and validity and cannot be held liable for any errors or omissions. Changes are periodically made to this book. You must consult your doctor or get professional medical advice before using any of the suggested remedies, techniques, or information in this book.

Upon using the information contained in this book, you agree to hold harmless the Author from and against any damages, costs, and expenses, including any legal fees potentially resulting from the application of any of the information provided by this guide. This disclaimer applies to any damages or injury caused by the use and application, whether directly or indirectly, of any advice or information presented, whether for breach of contract, tort, negligence, personal injury, criminal intent, or under any other cause of action.

You agree to accept all risks of using the information presented inside this book. You need to consult a professional medical practitioner in order to ensure you are both able and healthy enough to participate in this program.

Table of contents

Introduction

Over the past two decades, the prevalence of chronic kidney disease has been on the increase, while the mortality rate resulting from this disease is beginning to rise latently. The prevalence of chronic kidney disease (popular with its acronym- CKD) in 2017 was about 9% globally, which tells how much the disease is rapidly surging.

Between the early 90s' and 2017, the mortality rate from CKD has increased by 41.5%, making it the 12th leading cause of death globally. Notably, over a million deaths from cardiovascular disease have a link with chronic kidney disease.

There has not been a cure for kidney disease; however, it is possible to alleviate the situation and minimize damaging effects. A healthy dieting lifestyle and correct medication can help keep the kidneys healthier longer than anticipated.

An important aspect of revitalizing your kidney is eating well, i.e., eating what is right for your kidney health. Kidney-associated diseases are usually linked to unhealthy dieting and physical lifestyle. Eating healthy foods is essential in the treatment of kidney disease, as this will help

1

you feel better as well as helping you avoid complications of kidney disease such as bone disease, fluid overload, unhealthy weight loss, high blood potassium, and ultimately kidney failure.

This exposition is compiled to expose you to the reality of kidney disease in a preventive and corrective approach, which makes it a vital information source for every individual who values their kidneys health and overall wellbeing, as well as those who are battling with the reality of the kidney disease.

Chapter 1: The Organ-Kidney: All You Need To Know

The kidney description

Humans are created with a pair of kidneys (one on the right, the other on the left, with the spine in between them).

The kidneys are best described as reddish-brown bilaterally bean-shaped organs in the urinary system. The kidneys are located in the upper abdominal area against the back muscles. The left kidney is positioned a bit higher relative to the right kidney.

The kidney is an important member of the renal or urinary system and plays a vital role in osmoregulation. One of the primary roles of the kidney is to filter blood before sending it back to the heart, as well as helping the body to excrete waste as urine. The kidney is responsible for the transportation of urine to the bladder by the ureters. The urethra is responsible for taking the urine out of the body before passage through the perineum (in females), and then penis (in males).

This is why the nature/composition of your urine can tell so much about the health of your kidney.

What do the kidneys do- The functions of the kidneys
+ The roles of the kidney in urine formation

The sensors in the kidney cells help regulate the amount of water that is being excreted as urine, as well as the concentration of the electrolytes. For instance, when a person is dehydrated (loss of water) from exercise, the kidney will help retain as much water to keep the body hydrated, which then results in the urine being very concentrated. Whenever your urine is looking very colorful, this often tells you that you lack enough water. However, there could be more complications. On the other hand, when adequate water is present in your body, the urine is dilute, and hence becomes clear.
The biological mechanism above is regulated by a hormone called renin, which is produced in the kidney.

+ Kidney is a source of erythropoietin

Erythropoietin is a hormone, which stimulates the bone marrow to make red blood cells. The kidney does this by monitoring the oxygen concentration in the blood, and when the oxygen level declines, the erythropoietin levels increases, and more red blood cells is produced.

Other important functions and roles of the kidneys are:

+ Controlling blood pressure

+ It plays a role in activating vitamin D

+ Maintaining the overall fluid balance

+ Filtering and regulating minerals from the blood

Kidney possible health problems
The kidneys are usually exposed to various toxins in an attempt to filter waste (toxins) from the blood. Therefore, this vital role makes kidneys susceptible to various harmful conditions.
Some of these conditions include:

- Acidosis
- Acute nephritis
- Caliectasis
- Chronic kidney disease (CKD)
- Glomerulonephritis
- Kidney cysts
- Kidney failure
- Kidney stones
- Polycystic kidney disease

- Pyelonephritis
- Uremia
- Urinary tract infections

This is not an exhaustive list; there are other kidney-related conditions.
The focus here is on chronic kidney disease as well as kidney failure.

General risk factors of kidney diseases
A whole lot of factors and conditions can increase your risk of developing a kidney-related health condition. It is imperative to have a regular kidney test to ensure that they are functioning effectively, and if not, to what extent. The following health state triggers various kidney diseases:
✓ Diabetes
✓ Obesity
✓ High blood pressure
✓ Family history associated with kidney disease

Symptoms of kidney problems
There are specific symptoms of some kidney conditions; however, the following are the symptoms that can be associated with the most kidney problems:

✓ Foamy urine
✓ Itchy skin
✓ Fatigue
✓ Sleeplessness
✓ Muscle cramps
✓ Blood in urine
✓ Swelling (usually in the foot or ankle)
✓ Loss of appetite
✓ Inadequate or excessive urination

If you feel any of the symptoms, ensure to see your doctor for proper diagnosis through some kidney function tests.

Chapter 2: Chronic Kidney Disease (Ckd)

Chronic kidney disease (CKD) is a condition in which the effectiveness of the kidneys gradually slows down. The disease advances in stages, until it reaches the most severe- the end-stage renal disease (ESRD), also referred to as kidney failure. Chronic kidney disease can be reversed if it is caught early; modification of one's dietary lifestyle and use of proper medications can help slow down the advancement of the stages of chronic kidney disease.

The five stages of chronic kidney disease explained

The National Kidney Foundation (NKF) designed a guideline to assist doctors in the identification of each stage of kidney diseases, as each stage requires different tests and treatments. The parameter used is called the Glomerular Filtration Rate (GFR); this is the measure of the kidney function, as it used to determine a person's stage of kidney disease.

What the GFR measure is how effective is the kidney in the removal of serum creatinine from the blood. Creatinine is a metabolic waste product that comes from muscular activities. The higher the level of creatinine in the blood, the lower the GFR scores, and that means the effectiveness of the kidney drops as GFR scores drop, and vice versa.

The lower the GFR, the harmful it is to the kidneys

Below are the five stages of chronic kidney disease (CKD), and GFR for each stage:

GFR	Kidney Disease Stage	Interpretation
>90mL/min	Stage 1	Normal or high GFR (less than 100% effectiveness of kidney function)
60-89mL/min	Stage 2	Mild chronic kidney disease
45-59mL/min	Stage 3A	Moderate chronic kidney disease
30-44mL/min	Stage 3B	Moderate chronic kidney disease
15-29mL/min	Stage 4	Severe chronic kidney disease
<15mL/min	Stage 5	End-stage chronic kidney disease

From the table above, you can tell the stage of chronic kidney disease from the GFR result. However, each stage has its peculiar symptoms and possible treatment. Reversal is also possible if detected in time.

CKD: Stage 1 (GFR>90mL/min)
Most times, people in stage 1 of CKD are usually oblivious of the fact that their kidneys are not functioning at its best. At this stage, the kidney does a good job but will not function at 100%; this is why there are usually no symptoms to tell that the kidneys are getting damaged.

Most times, people who are in stage 1 find out when they are being tested for another condition such as high blood pressure or diabetes, which are the leading culprit behind the CKD.

Symptoms of stage 1 CKD
Except for being tested, it could be very difficult to know you are in stage 1 CKD. However, the symptoms could include:
✓   Creatinine or urea in the blood rising higher above normal levels.
✓   Blood or protein in the urine.

Treatment for stage 1 CKD
Discovering that you are in stage 1 CKD is the best way to address chronic kidney disease. This can be done by regularly testing for protein in the urine and serum creatinine, which can tell if the kidney damage is progressing.

When you are diagnosed with stage 1 CKD, ensure you adhere to the following health tips:

•   Eat a healthy diet, which should include a variety of grains (whole grains), vegetables, and fresh fruits.
•   Ensure that your diet is low in saturated fat and cholesterol.
•   Avoid salty food, use less salt in your meal.
•   Limit your intake of processed and refined foods, especially those high in sugar.
•   Keep your blood sugar level under control.
•   Engage in physical exercises regularly.
•   Quit smoking and excessive alcohol.
•   Most importantly, have regular checkups to measure your GFR.

CKD: Stage 2 (GFR= 60-89mL/min)
Just as in stage 1 CKD, stage 2 CKD has similar indications and symptoms. This is a mild chronic kidney disease, and it might be difficult to know that one is in stage 2 CKD, as there are usually no obvious symptoms.

Symptoms of stage 2 CKD

Same as stage 1 CKD

Treatment for stage 1 CKD

Refer to stage 1 CKD.
CKD: Stage 3 (GFR= 59-30mL/min)
This signifies moderate kidney damage. The stage is divided into two:
Stage 3A (with GFR between 45-59mL/min);

Stage 3B (with GFR between 30-44 mL/min)

In stage 3 CKD, the function of the kidney continues to decline, hence leading to waste build up in the blood, consequently resulting in a condition known as uremia. Stage 3 CKD usually comes with complications such as high blood pressure and/or anemia.

Symptoms of stage 3 CKD

The following symptoms may begin to manifest at stage 3 CKD:

✓ Urination begins to appear in foamy brown or dark orange or red if it contains blood.
✓ Kidney pain felt in the back.
✓ Sleeplessness resulting from muscle cramps.
✓ Fatigue

✓   Swelling (edema)

✓   Shortness of breath

Line of action

When diagnosed with stage 3 CKD, the patient should see a nephrologist. A nephrologist is a doctor who specializes in treating kidney disease. The nephrologist gathers as much information as possible from the patient, perform a lab test to proffer the best treatment advice.

Aside from seeing a nephrologist, someone in stage 3 should consider consulting a dietitian. The reason why it is important to see a dietitian is that diet is an important aspect of treating any kidney disease. The dietitian will review the lab results and then recommend a proper meal plan.

What to eat and what not to

As previously stated, diet plays a vital role in helping to maintain the overall health of the kidney. A healthy diet should follow the following guidelines:

- Consumption of whole grains, fruits, and vegetables
- Eat high-quality protein and potassium diet if blood levels are above normal
- Lower calcium and phosphorus consumption
- Limiting the consumption of saturated fats
- Cutting back on carbohydrates for diabetic patients
- Lower sodium diet by cutting out highly processed foods (esp. patients with high blood pressure or fluid retention)

Note: Always consult with a registered renal dietitian, because as the stages of CKD change, the diet is expected to change as well.

Stage 3 CKD and medications

Most patients who develop CKD usually have diabetes or high blood pressure. Most times, a doctor will likely prescribe the same drugs both for diabetic patients, and those with high blood pressure. Ensure to ask the doctor about the complications with the prescribed drugs and use them exactly as prescribed.

Aside from medications, healthy activities like regular exercises should be encouraged. At the same time, unhealthy practices such as smoking should be avoided to prolong the health of the kidney.

CKD: Stage 4 (GFR= 15-30 mL/min)
A person with stage 4 CKD is in the advanced stage of kidney damage. At this stage, dialysis or a kidney transplant is very much likely. (More on dialysis and kidney transplant in the subsequent chapters).
At this stage, the kidney function declines progressively and less effective than stages 3, 2, and 1. This results in complications of kidney diseases such as high blood pressure, bone disease, anemia, and other cardiovascular diseases due to a build-up of toxic waste in the blood.
Symptoms of stage 4 CKD

•   Nausea/vomiting
•   Bad breathe resulting from urea build-up in the blood
•   Loss of appetite
•   Numbness in the toes or fingers
•   Difficulty in concentration (focus)
Also include symptoms from stage CKD

Line of action

People in stage 4 CKD are expected to schedule a meeting with the doctor at least once in three months. Seeing a nephrologist is a must at this stage. At this stage, the nephrologist might prepare the patient for a dialysis session or a kidney transplant depending on the severity of the condition.

Diet and stage 4 CKD

The diet guidelines are quite similar to stage 3.

• Reduce protein intake to avoid excessive protein waste build-up
• Consumption of whole grains, fruits, and vegetables
• Eat high-quality protein and potassium diet if blood levels are above normal
• Lower calcium and phosphorus consumption
• Limiting the consumption of saturated fats
• Cutting back on carbohydrates for diabetic patients
• Lower sodium diet by cutting out highly processed foods (esp. patients with high blood pressure or fluid retention)

The treatment options at stage 4 CKD

At stage 4 CKD, the treatment options are usually going for dialysis or kidney transplant. Let's examine the options clearly:

1.   Hemodialysis

A dialysis machine removes an amount of the patient's blood through an artificial membrane called a dialyzer or artificial kidney to filter out toxins that the kidneys can no longer remove. Then the filtered blood is returned to the blood. This treatment can be done in a patient's home but with the help of a care partner.

2.   Peritoneal dialysis (PD)

Peritoneal dialysis (PD) uses the lining of the abdominal cavity as the dialysis filter to rid the body of waste and to balance electrolyte levels.

3.   Kidney transplant

This is the most effective treatment of chronic kidney disease, and it is usually the last resort. It does not require diet restriction, unlike for those on regular CKD treatment or those on hemodialysis or peritoneal dialysis.
Please note that the National Kidney Foundation (NKF) recommends that dialysis should begin when GFR drops to 15 % or less.

CKD: Stage 5 (GFR <15 %)

At stage 5 CKD, a person is said to have reached end-stage renal disease (ESRD). At this stage, the kidneys are deemed to have lost nearly all of its effective functions. The introduction of dialysis or a kidney transplant is inevitable to keep the patient alive.

Symptoms of stage 5 CKD

The symptoms associated with stage 5 CKD include:
✓ Production of little or no urine
✓ Loss of appetite
✓ Nausea or vomiting
✓ Headaches
✓ Restlessness
✓ Unable to focus and concentrate
✓ Itching
✓ Muscle cramps
✓ Swelling
✓ Change in skin color and increased skin pigmentation

Line of action

At stage 5 CKD, an immediate visit to the nephrologist is compulsory. The doctor will help you decide on the type of treatment that will work best for you.

Treatment options
Dialysis has proved effective, as most people tend to get better once they begin the dialysis session. However, if there is no much improvement, then a kidney transplant would be the last resort.

If you wish to have a kidney transplant, you can discuss it with your nephrologist. Then your nephrologist will explain the process to you and the cost implications.

Stage 5 CKD and diet
As soon as the dialysis begins, your dietitian will enlighten you on what to eat and what to avoid. The type of diet that your dietitian chooses will be based on the type of dialysis treatment you choose and your specific dietary requirement.

A healthy diet for stage 5 CKD may include:

•   Grains, fruits, and vegetables (limit whole grains, and fruits and vegetables high in potassium or phosphorus)
•   Decreasing calcium intake
•   Diet low in saturated fat and cholesterol

- Limiting consumption of sodium especially in refined and processed food

Your dietitian will give more recommendations based on your individual needs.

Living with kidney disease
There is no proven permanent cure for kidney disease, but it is possible to stop its progress or slow down its damage. To keep the kidneys healthier for a longer period, it is vital to adhere to the correct treatment as prescribed by your doctor and adjusting to some behavioral lifestyle.

Chapter 3: The Kidney Failure

When the kidneys fail, it means they have stopped working well enough for survival except with the aid of dialysis or a kidney transplant. Kidney failure is also known as an end-stage renal disease (ESRD), which is the last stage of chronic kidney disease (CKD).

Treatment of the underlying disease causing kidney failure can help restore the kidneys' functions to normal. In some cases, kidney failure may be progressive and may be irreversible.

One of the best ways to prevent chronic kidney disease, which progresses into kidney failure, is a lifelong effort to control high blood pressure and diabetes.

As we age, it is normal for the kidneys functions to decrease. Still, a rapid decrease in functionality of the kidneys is detrimental.
If the kidneys fail completely, the options could be dialysis or a kidney transplant. Fortunately, if one of the kidneys fails or is diseased, it can be removed. In contrast, the remaining kidney may continue to have normal renal functions.
What causes kidney failure?

Kidney failure could occur from a chronic disease that causes the kidneys to stop functioning or from an acute situation that injures the kidneys.

Diabetes remains the major culprit behind the cause of kidney failure, while high blood pressure follows. Meanwhile, other causes of kidney failure include urinary tract problems, autoimmune diseases such as lupus, polycystic kidney disease, genetic disease, nephritic syndrome, and so on.

In acute renal failure, the kidneys could stop working suddenly (this can occur within 48 hours). The common causes of this could be the illegal use of drugs/drug abuse, heart attack, urinary tract problems, and insufficient blood flow to the kidneys. Acute renal failure is not always permanent and can be reversed with treatments.

The following can result in acute kidney failure:

•   Obstruction of the renal artery or vein resulting in abnormal blood flow to and from the kidney
•   Poor intake of fluids
•   Low blood volume

- Loss of excessive body fluid resulting from vomiting, diarrhea, fever, or intense sweating
- Medications such as diuretics may cause excessive water loss, other medications toxic to the kidney include but not limited to:
- Non-steroidal anti-inflammatory drugs
- Antibiotics such as aminoglycosides gentamicin
- Iodine-containing medications

Below are the post-renal causes of kidney failure:

Post-renal causes of kidney failure refer to factors that affect the outflow of urine and consequently having a backwash effect on the kidneys.

- Obstruction of the bladder or the ureters

Much pressure will be formed on the kidneys as it continues to produce urine. When the pressure is high enough that the kidneys cannot resist, the kidneys are damaged.

- Abdomen tumors (obstructing the ureters)
- Prostate cancer

- Kidney stone

Other conditions that can cause kidney failure include:

- Rhabdomyolysis: This refers to a significant breakdown of muscle in the body, leading to the clogging of the kidneys filtering system by the damaged muscle fibers. The possible causes of muscle injuries/breakdown could be trauma, burns, and some high cholesterol medications.

The symptoms of kidney failure
When the kidneys start to fail, you may notice one or more of the following symptoms:

- Acidosis
- Anemia
- Edema (generalized swelling)
- Excessive or inadequate urination
- Fatal heart rhythm disturbance
- Fever
- Hyperkalemia (high blood potassium)
- Itching
- Lethargy
- Loss of appetite
- Muscle cramps
- Nausea/vomiting

- Nose bleed
- Rash
- Sleeplessness
- Weakness

If you notice one or more of any symptoms above, it could be a sign of a serious kidney problem. Contact your doctor immediately.

What procedures and tests diagnose kidney failure?

Urine tests are usually ordered to detect the presence of abnormal cells, amount of protein, or the concentration of electrolytes, and this information can give a hint on the nature of the kidney but not an affirmative test for kidney failure.

To diagnose kidney failure, blood test such as GFR needs to be executed to measure the build-up of waste products in the blood.

Other types of test can diagnose the type of kidney failure; example includes:

- Abdominal ultrasound
- Kidney biopsy

Chapter 4: Kidney Dialysis Or Transplant

Whenever kidney failure occurs, the renal function ceases and could lead to a more consequential outcome and, ultimately, death. However, with dialysis or kidney transplant, the renal functions can be restored.

Dialysis

Dialysis cleanses the waste products in the body by the use of filter systems. Dialysis is done in an attempt to help the kidneys to perform its primary functions, which is the filtering of waste products in the blood. Dialysis treatments usually occur thrice a week.

The National Kidney Foundation (NKF) recommends that dialysis should begin when GFR drops to 15 % or less.

There are two types of dialysis:

A. Hemodialysis

This process of dialysis uses a machine filter (dialyzer) or artificial kidney to remove waste products of metabolism and eradicate excess salt and water in an attempt to balance other electrolytes in the body.

Blood is removed from the body, and it is made to flow through a tube into the dialyzer, where it is passed next to a filter membrane. A specialized chemical solution is formulated to draw impurities from the blood via the filter membrane.

B. Peritoneal dialysis

Peritoneal dialysis uses the abdominal cavity lining as the dialysis filter instead of a machine dialyzer as in hemodialysis. It aims to rid the body of waste and balance the electrolyte level. It is a process that is carried out by a surgeon.

As there are benefits for each type of dialysis, so also are complications for each. Therefore, it is not always the case that a patient can choose which type of dialysis they want, the treatment depends on the decision made on the patient's illness and their past medical history, as well as other health issues attached to the kidney problem. The nephrologist will proffer the best option after discussing it with the patient.

Note: When the kidneys no longer function, dialysis could be the lifesaver. However, patients may live many years on dialysis but could still pass out from other underlying and associated illnesses.

What is life like on dialysis?

The start of dialysis is like a new life, which comes with adjusting some aspects of your life, from managing a new set of diets to staying on medications, finding new ways to enjoy your daily activities, and so on. You don't have to worry; you will adapt in time.

Is a kidney transplant an option?

Kidney transplant is usually the more suitable option when kidney failure is non-reversible.
The nephrologist will help determine if the patient is an appropriate candidate. Then they will proceed to contact an organ transplant center to evaluate the patient suitability for this treatment. You might be lucky to find a family member with compatible tissue type and willing to donate a kidney. Most times, it boils down to being placed on the organ transplant list regulated by the United Network of Organ Sharing (UNOS).
Complications with a kidney transplant
As with any medical operations, there is a risk of bleeding and infection from the openings.

The body can attempt to reject the transplanted kidney, and it might even fail to work.

If the kidney transplant fails, then the alternative is to repeat another kidney transplant or return to dialysis.

However, kidney transplant gives a better chance of quality life than dialysis.

Chapter 5: The Rules Of Renal Diet

Aside from medications, diet is an important consideration for those battling with any stage of chronic kidney disease, acute or chronic kidney failure. Following a strict diet plan as directed by a dietitian can lessen the accumulation of toxins.

When the kidney is in an impaired state, the kidney cannot easily perform some of its functions, such as removing excess water, salt, or potassium from the blood. With this in mind, food high in potassium salt should be consumed with care.

A dietitian can help you decide what type of diet may be helpful and what food might be inappropriate for your kidneys health.
Detoxifying the kidney
Detoxifying the kidneys is an effective way of prolonging and preserving the health of the kidneys.

The following fruits/herbs/plants are known to be effective in cleansing the kidneys:

✓ Apple cider vinegar
✓ Basil
✓ Beet juice
✓ Cranberry juice
✓ Dandelion
✓ Dates
✓ Ginger
✓ Kidney beans
✓ Lemon juice
✓ Pumpkin seeds
✓ Smoothies
✓ Turmeric
✓ Watermelon

Meeting my nutritional needs with kidney disease

Having kidney disease comes with diet-restriction, and you might be worried about meeting your nutritional needs. It is not as difficult as you might think, it is all about knowing what you should avoid, what you should reduce or remove completely from your diet.

Practicing portion control is a very good way of restricting some minerals and nutrients intake. For instance, a high-protein diet can cause your diseased kidney to work too hard; therefore, you should take a smaller portion of protein in your meal. Also, be aware that your protein restriction depends on your stage of kidney disease.

Is it safe to eat out managing kidney disease?
At first, it may look challenging, but you can find kidney-friendly foods at some American restaurants. You just have to inform them of your condition, as they are aware there are people with kidney disease who rely on a strict renal diet.

Follow these simple guidelines if you are eating out of the house:

✓   Always request no added salt
✓   Choose dishes with steamed rice instead of fried.
✓   Don't add sauces such as soy sauce, and fish sauce into your meal.

Chapter 6: Potassium Diet And Kidney Disease

Potassium is one of the electrolytes that the kidneys try to balance its concentration in the blood. When the renal functions diminish, the kidney's ability to regulate potassium drops significantly, and this results in a high concentration of potassium in the blood

A high level of potassium develops slowly over weeks or months, which usually leads to feelings of nausea or fatigue. Again, some medications dedicated to treating kidney diseases are also capable of raising potassium, which is another problem. Spike in potassium concentration in the blood could lead to a condition known as hyperkalemia. It is a condition that requires immediate medical care, with symptoms such as chest pain, difficulty in breathing, or heart palpitations.

Minimizing potassium build-up in diet

Some foods are high in potassium, while some are low. Aside from doing thorough research on foods that are low in potassium, you should learn to read the nutritional labels on your packaged food items.

It is possible to get a spike in potassium level even when you consume a low-potassium diet but in large quantities. In a simpler term, even if a diet is low in potassium, it doesn't mean it should be eaten in large quantities to avoid a spike in potassium concentration.

Below is a list of food low in potassium:
✓ Apples
✓ Berries (blueberries and strawberries)
✓ Broccoli
✓ Cauliflower
✓ Egg white
✓ Eggplant
✓ Green beans
✓ Pineapple
✓ White bread
✓ White pasta
✓ White rice

Note: Foods are considered to be low in potassium if they contain less than 200 milligrams (or exactly) per serving. This is why quantity matters as well.

High-potassium foods
The following foods are proven to contain over 200 mg potassium per serving. They should be avoided when you are battling with kidney disease or kidney failure.

✓ Apricots

- ✓ Avocados
- ✓ Bananas
- ✓ Beef
- ✓ Brussels sprouts
- ✓ Cantaloupe
- ✓ Chicken
- ✓ Dried apricots
- ✓ Lentils
- ✓ Low-sodium cheese
- ✓ Milk
- ✓ Nuts
- ✓ Oranges
- ✓ Potatoes
- ✓ Prunes
- ✓ Pumpkin
- ✓ Raisins
- ✓ Spinach
- ✓ Split peas
- ✓ Tomatoes (juice and sauce)
- ✓ Yogurt

Note: Depending on your kidney state, you might be able to include some amounts of foods high in potassium in your diet without harm. Discuss with your dietitian and ask questions about your diet options.

How to leach potassium vegetables

Sometime you might be tempted to cook a dish with a high-potassium vegetable, and you don't wish to replace it with another; there is a solution. You can leach some of the potassium from the vegetable.

The National Kidney Foundation (NKF) recommended a step-wise approach to leaching beets, winter squash, carrots, rutabagas, and potatoes. Below is the description:

• After peeling the vegetable, place in cold water to avoid darkening
• Slice the vegetable into one-eight inch-thick parts
• In warm water, rinse for about 10-15 seconds
• Soak the cut piece in warm water for about two hours to four hours
• For a few seconds, rinse the vegetable under warm water again
• Cook the vegetable with a water volume of about five times the amount of vegetables.

Complete

How to reduce the potassium level in canned foods
Canned fruits and vegetables are known to be a route of exposure to high potassium intake; this is why it advisable to go for fresh or frozen fruits and vegetables. The potassium canned

product leaches into the liquid content in the can, therefore using this liquid in your meal can cause a significant increase in your potassium levels.

However, if you are considering the canned version, then you must do yourself some good by leaching the potassium off the canned product, by draining the juice and discarding it. The canned food should also be rinsed with water before use.

How much potassium is safe in my diet?
People with kidney disease are expected to restrict their potassium intake below 2,000mg daily. This is why it is important to check your potassium level through a simple blood test. There are three levels of potassium concentration in the blood as given below:

- Safe zone: 3.5 to 5.0 mmol/L
- Caution zone: 5.1 to 6.0 mmol/L
- Danger zone: 6.0 mmol/L or higher

Your doctor can help you determine your daily potassium intake limit from the test result while maintaining the highest level of nutrition possible.

Chapter 7: Tips For Healthy Kidneys

The kidneys are one of the most vital organs in the body, and when they are unhealthy; it can break down the whole body system completely and could lead to death. However, you can keep the kidneys healthy by following the tips below:

Stay hydrated

It is more harmful to drink inadequate water than drinking too much water. However, drinking plenty of water helps your kidney performs its functions well. Water helps in dilution; therefore, this aids the kidneys in removing toxins with ease.

Therefore consider the healthy practice of drinking enough water, if not for anything, but the health of your kidneys.

Exercise

One of the risk factors of chronic kidney disease is high blood pressure. It is proven that regular exercise can help reduce blood pressure.

Therefore, inculcate the habit of exercising every day, even if it will require you to take a walk.

Cut out extra salt

Eating too much salty food makes it harder for the kidney to function properly. One of the easiest routes to eating salty meals is processed foods, which usually have a lot of salt added. Therefore try to swap such a diet for fresh fruits, vegetables, nuts, and low-fat meals.

Use medications with caution

Regular intake of certain over-the-counter medications can be harmful to your kidney. Regular use of non-steroidal anti-inflammatory drugs is one of those medications you should be cautious of as their effects on the kidney over time can be detrimental.Discuss other alternatives with your doctors if you have a condition that requires managing pain.

Chapter 8: Your Kidney And Its Core Functions Explained

Your kidneys are a pair of 4 -5 inches bean-shaped organs located at both sides of your spine and like most organs in the body, they carry the all-important function of eliminating waste from your bloodstream and body.

Other equally important functions the kidneys carry out include:

- Regulating your overall fluid balance and eliminating any excess as urine.

- Producing some hormones that regulate the functions of a few other organs.

- Regulating the functions of your red blood cells.

- Eliminating drugs or toxins from your system through urine.

- Maintaining your body's salt, potassium, and acids balance.

Your Kidney Makeup

Each of your kidneys is made up of close to a million nephrons all functioning to filter your blood and eliminate waste and excess water from the blood.

Each nephron contains a filtering unit of little blood vessels that carry out this job of filtering. These nephrons are constantly working as the 1-1.5 gallons of blood in your system gets filtered about 40 times a day!

Why Your Kidneys are So Important

Being one of the five vital organs in the human body alongside your heart, brain, lungs, and liver, your kidneys are very much needed and their health should be closely guarded.

However, while most people get born with two functioning kidneys, you only really need just one to live a healthy life. People who have lost one kidney, either as a result of it getting damaged or by donating it to save a life, find they can live healthy, quality lives with very little to no complications.

If, on the other hand, this last kidney gets damaged, a condition that is known as Chronic Kidney Disease (CKD), then your body goes into what is medically termed uremia, a health complication where your bloodstream gets filled with the waste, toxins, and excess water that didn't get filtered out. Uremia is characterized by symptoms such as

- Extreme tiredness and fatigue
- Nausea and vomiting
- Low to no appetite
- Headache
- Leg cramps or numbness
- Weakness
- Weight loss
- High blood pressure
- Swellings in the feet or ankles
- Trouble concentrating

It is also a potentially fatal condition, however, while CKD can't be treated, its progression can be halted before it develops into uremia.

Knowing All There is to Know about Chronic Kidney Disease (CKD)
As earlier mentioned, Chronic Kidney Disease occurs when your kidneys become damaged and can no longer filter blood like they are supposed to.

This disease, however, does not just happen out of the blues, but progresses over some time through a series of stages and symptoms. As the disease progresses (if not caught in time and effectively managed), there's a gradual loss in your kidney functions. With this loss, waste, toxins, and excess water can't get filtered out if the blood builds up, possibly leading to other health complications where you become very sick.

What Causes Chronic Kidney Disease?

Several factors have been known to cause or contribute to the progression of CKD, however, two main factors are diabetes and high blood pressure as both are responsible for up to 70% of all CKD cases.

Most cases of diabetes lead to chronic kidney disease. When the sugar level in your bloodstream rises to such an unhealthy high, it causes damage to organs in the body, including the kidneys.

High blood pressure, on the other hand, has been linked to CKD in that the pressure at which the blood pumps through the blood vessels become so forceful, it exerts too much pressure on the walls of these vessels. If not properly managed, high blood pressure could lead to CKD and other heart-related complications like heart attack and stroke.
Other well-known causes of chronic kidney disease include:

- Untreated or recurrent urinary tract infection.

- Lupus

- Polycystic kidney disease

- Infection

- Lead poisoning

- Alport syndrome (a genetic condition where the blood vessels in the kidney become destroyed)

- Renal artery stenosis

- Hemolytic uremic syndrome (where red blood cells become destroyed and negatively impact or block the kidney filtering system).

Stages of Chronic Kidney Disease
As earlier said, chronic kidney disease doesn't just occur but does so over some time and this is good because it does afford the patient the chance to prolonged life.

With the early discovery, you can begin treatment to halt its progression to the next stage using the right combination of medicine, lifestyle habits, and dietary change.

The National Kidney Foundation (NKF) has identified five stages or progression of kidney disease, with each having its set of symptoms and level of severity.

The Chronic Kidney Disease stage is determined based on the individual's Glomerular Filtration Rate (GFR).

The glomerular filtration rate is the best way to determine how healthy or otherwise a kidney is and is calculated using your gender, age, race, and your body's creatinine.

The five stages of kidney disease are:

Stage One (GFR > 90 ml/min)

With stage one, your GFR levels are normal or high (above 90), however, there is some evidence of slight kidney damage, although not enough to impact the regular kidney functions.

Stage one of CKD is usually regarded as not too serious and you can halt the disease progression at this stage by making some lifestyle or dietary changes.

Stage Two (GFR = 60-89 mL/min)

Stage two is regarded as mild CKD and also presents with very little to no symptoms, so it's also very likely to miss the disease presence altogether.

In this stage, your GFR reduces and is somewhat in the vicinity of 60-89.
A lot of the people who find out they have stage two CKD chance upon this information when being tested for other health complications like high blood pressure or diabetes.

Management and treatment of stage two CKD usually involve dietary changes which include:

- Limiting salt and sodium intake.
- Reducing processed foods or foods high in sugar.
- Opting for a low-fat and low-cholesterol diet.
- Working with a dietician to get the right protein need for your body.
- Upping your vitamin and mineral intake as recommended by your doctor.

- Getting the right weight, if you happen to be overweight.
- Including whole grains, fruits, and veggies in your diet.
- Exercising regularly.
- Keeping your blood sugar level balanced.
- Monitoring your blood pressure.

Stage Three (GFR 30-59)

With stage three the kidneys are moderately damaged and aren't as healthy as they should be. Stage three chronic kidney disease is further classified into two stages:

- Stage 3A (GFR 45-59) and
- Stage 3B (GFR 30-44)

Stage three CKD is usually regarded as serious as your kidney's ability to filter out wastes and toxins reduces, making these toxins build up in the blood, leading to uremia.

A stage three CKD patient is also highly at risk of other health complications related to CKD such as anemia and hypertension.

Symptoms you can expect to see with stage three CKD include shortness of breath, changes in your urine colour ranging from dark orange to brown or red (bloodstained), fatigue, fluid retention, swellings in the legs, pain in your kidney region or lower back, and difficulty sleeping.

Management for stage three CKD typically involves going on the right diet as advised by your dietician and undergoing the right medications as prescribed by your nephrologists.

It should be noted that while it is strongly recommended you embark on the right medication and diet to halt the disease progression, over half of all stage three kidney disease cases still progress to stages four and five over several years.

The good news though, is that life expectancy for people living with stage three CKD is still somewhat on the high side when the right diet and lifestyle habits are maintained. Men aged 40 and above diagnosed with kidney disease can still live for 24 years while women in the same position can still live for up to 28 years.
Other ways to extend your life quality, expectancy and to also slow the progression to stage four include:

- Exercising for upward of 30 minutes at least five days a week.

- Including lots of fruits, veggies, and whole grains in your diet.

- Eliminating smoking cigarettes or the use of other tobacco products.

- Cutting down on your intake of processed sugar and sodium.

- Cutting down on your intake of saturated fat and cholesterol.

- Carrying out regular checks on your sugar level and blood pressure.

Stage Four (GFR 15-30 mL/min)

This is the last stage of chronic kidney disease before the disease progresses to kidney failure. At this stage, the patient will begin to show noticeable signs of the disease and be visibly sick.

The kidneys are severely damaged at this stage and the patient will need a transplant shortly.

This is also the stage where the patient likely begins to experience other health complications like anemia, high blood pressure, bone problems, and heart-related diseases.

Symptoms of stage four CKD include fluid retention, fatigue, changes in your urine colour, kidney pain felt at your lower back, nausea, and vomiting, a loss in appetite, numbness or a tingling feeling in your fingers and toes, bad breath, and difficulties concentrating.

Like stage three, stage four CKD can also be managed to give you a better quality of life and to also slow down its progression to stage five.
Your doctor will usually recommend the right combination of treatment, diet, and lifestyle changes for your case.

Some treatment options for stage four kidney disease include:

1. Hemodialysis

A treatment plan where waste and excess water get filtered from your body using a machine. A small portion of your blood gets extracted, filtered, and returned to your body.

2. Peritoneal Dialysis (PD)

Peritoneal Dialysis (PD) is dialysis that can be carried out at home by the patient, often without medical assistance or supervision.

3. Kidney Transplant

An option that could come in if the disease progresses to stage five.
Other treatment options for stage four kidney disease include eating a healthy diet, limiting your salt intake to less than 6g daily, quitting unhealthy lifestyle habits, and maintaining the right weight.

Stage Five (GFR Less than 15)

This is the last and advanced stage of kidney disease and here, the kidneys have lost most of their functions and can no longer filter the blood.

To stay alive, the patient would have to begin ongoing dialysis or get a kidney transplant.

Some symptoms of this end-stage CKD or kidney failure include:

- Little or no appetite
- Nausea or vomiting
- Fatigue
- Inability to concentrate
- Headache
- Producing very little to no urine
- Swellings around the ankles
- Numbness or tingling in the heads or feet
- A noticeable change in your skin tone or colour
- Muscle cramps

The Three Electrolyte Components in Your Body and Their Functions

- Sodium

Sodium is a mineral and electrolyte that's essential for the body's normal functioning and around 85% of it can be found in the blood and lymph fluids.

This mineral carries out be following functions:

- Fluid balancing (maintaining the ideal water balance in the body).
- Regulates blood volume and blood pressure.
- Regulates nerve and muscle functions.

- Potassium

Potassium, as a nutrient, works hand-in-hand with sodium. One of its main functions is to help your nerves and muscles contract.

 It also carries out others like helping nutrients to move into cells and wastes out of it and helping your heartbeat stay regular.

- Phosphorus

The man function of phosphorus is for bone and teeth formation. However, it also carries out other functions as it helps the body produce proteins essential for the growth, maintenance, and repair of cells and tissues as well as determine how the body uses fats and carbohydrates.

20 Foods to Avoid When Diagnosed of Chronic Kidney Disease

Dietary needs for people with kidney disease differ. People with the beginning stage of kidney disease, also known as stage 1 kidney disease, have a dietary restriction that is different from patients on stages four or five.

Your doctor or healthcare provider is usually charged with determining what your diet should be at this stage you are in.

This dietary restriction, also called a renal diet, is geared towards ensuring you maintain the best health possible. it will ensure your kidneys function at the best possible state while helping to reduce the amount of waste and creatinine buildup in your bloodstream.

Some nutrients your doctor will recommend you reduce in varying degrees include:

 - Sodium (limiting to less than 2000 MG daily)

- Potassium (also limited to less than 2000 MG daily)

- Phosphorus (reduced to within the range of 800 to 1000 MG daily)

-    Protein (reduced in early-stage kidney disease, but increased in later stage renal failure)

 Some food you should avoid include the following :

1. Avocados (avoided due to their high deposit of potassium)

2. Canned food (avoided for their high sodium deposits)

3. Whole-wheat bread (avoided for its high phosphorus and potassium deposits)

4. Brown rice (taken only on a controlled basis as it also has high phosphorus and potassium deposits).

5. Bananas (high potassium content)

6. Dairy products (high in phosphorus and potassium)

7. Oranges (high in potassium)

8. Processed meat (high in sodium and protein)

9. Apricots (avoided due to their high potassium deposit)

10. All kinds of potatoes (high in potassium, but can be taken if soaked this reduces some of the potassium deposit)

11 . Tomatoes (high in potassium)

12. Spinach and beet greens (high in potassium)

13. Dates and raisins (high in potassium)

14. Chips and crackers (high in sodium and potassium)
15. Sodas

16. Ice cream

17. Plantains

18. Corn and products made out of corn like corn flakes and chips

19. White rice

20. Peas

21. Lentils

Foods you should include in your renal diet for their low-to-moderate potassium and sodium content include:

1. Red bell peppers

2. Cabbage

3. Cauliflower

4. Garlic
5. Onions

6. Apples

7. Berries: blueberries, raspberries, cranberries, and strawberries.

8. Cherries

9. Red grapes

10. Egg whites

11. Fish

12. Olive oil

13. Sea bass

14. Buckwheat

15. Skinless chicken

16. Radish

17. Turnips

18. Pineapples

19. Bulgur

20. Arugula

21. Macadamia nuts

22. Fish with high Omega-3 fatty acids like salmon, mackerel, sardines, and herring

23. Kale

24. Cranberry juice

25. Wine

26. Water

What is Renal Diet: All You Need to Know

You should already have an idea what a renal diet is (if you didn't previously), but just so there is no confusion, here's a really simple definition of what a renal diet is.

A renal diet is one that's suitable for people with kidney disease. It is one with a low to moderate amount of sodium, potassium, and protein and also emphasizes the need to limit the amount of liquid you consume daily and to take in high-quality protein.

Importance of a Renal Diet

For people with kidney disease, taking in too much of a few nutrients (phosphorus, potassium, sodium, and even calcium) could be detrimental to their health. This is where a renal diet comes in.

The renal diet is a super-easy way for CKD patients to monitor the intake of nutrients like sodium potassium and phosphorus.

In summary, here are a few ways a renal diet benefits CKD patients:

1. It promotes regular kidney function, giving you a better quality of life.

2. It's slow the progression of the disease from the stage it's currently at to the next.

Some Quick Facts about Going on a Renal Diet

1. It's always strongly recommended you work with a renal dietitian for your meal plan as they have extensive knowledge and expert ideas on the topic.

2. A renal guide emphasizing limiting protein, however a patient at the end stage of kidney failure would need more high-quality protein.

3. The daily phosphorus intake on a renal diet is usually limited to 1000 mg for maximum health. It is strongly recommended you avoid these high-phosphorus foods; chocolate, red beans, black beans, white beans, whole or unrefined grain, and dark coloured sodas. Too much phosphorus is harmful when you have kidney disease, however, you need some quantity of it daily to maintain a regular/normal water balance in your body. These are the phosphorus that should be taken in moderate quantity; dairy, poultry, and eat.

4. Sodium as a nutrient is essential for your normal bodily functions and also serves to regulate the fluid balance in your system.

Sodium is mostly found in table salt, which makes reducing or limiting it in your diet a little easier.

If you plan on reducing your salt intake here are a few ways you can achieve this:

- Avoid cooking with salt or use as little salt as possible
- When shopping check each food label to ensure each item does not exceed over 300mg sodium for each serving.
- Cut out of your diet completely, food like canned soup, sausages, bacon, bologna, ham, salted crackers, chips, and instant noodles are known to have high sodium content.

- Avoid other salt alternatives.

Renal Diet Menus

Recipe One

- Cottage cheese pancakes with whipped cream and one egg white.
- A cup of coffee or tea with creamer (optional)

Recipe Two

- 1 Sausage
- 1 Scrambled egg
- 2 Teaspoons baked beans
- 3 Toasts

Recipe Three

- Porridge oats (35g)
- Full-fat milk (if trying to gain weight otherwise substitute with skimmed milk) (200ml)
- ½ Grated apples
- A dash of ground cinnamon

Recipe Four

Turkey Breakfast Burrito

Ingredients
- 4 Eggs (beaten, scrambled)
- 4 6-inch flour burrito shells
- ⅛ Cup granola oil
- ½ Pound ground chicken
- ⅛ Cup onions (diced)
- ⅛ Cup fresh bell peppers
- 1 Tablespoon fresh scallions (chopped)
- 1 Tablespoon fresh cilantro (chopped)
- 1 Tablespoon seeded Jalapeñõ peppers
- ¼ Teaspoon paprika (smoked)
- ¼ Teaspoon chili powder

-½ Cup Monterey Jack and Cheddar cheese (shredded)

Directions

1) Place a sauté pan on medium heat with half the oil. Pour in onions, peppers, scallions, meatloaf, and cilantro and allow sauté until it becomes translucent. Add the spices and turn off the heat.

2) Pour the oil left into another pan and also place on medium heat. Pour the scrambled eggs.

3) Put the same amount of the meatloaf mixture and veggies in the burrito shells, fold and serve.

Recipe Five

Spicy Tofu Scrambler
Ingredients

-½ Cup tofu (firm)
- ⅛ Cup red bell pepper (chopped)
- ⅛ Cup green bell pepper
- ½ Teaspoon olive oil
- ½ Teaspoon onion powder

- ⅛ Teaspoon garlic powder
- 1 Clove garlic (minced)
- A pinch of salt

Directions

1) Pour olive oil into a non-stick skillet and place on medium heat. Sauté bell peppers and garlic.

2) Rinse tofu then crumble into the skillet.

3) Stir in the remaining ingredients.

4) Reduce heat and allow it to cook for 15 minutes or until it turns a light golden brown.

5) Take off heat and serve.

Renal Diet Recipes for a Diabetic

Recipe One

Easy Breakfast
Ingredients
- 1 Cup Rice Krispies Cereal
- 4 Ounces Nondairy creamer
- 4 Ounces unsweetened grape juice
- ½ English muffin
- 1 Teaspoon fruit jam

- 1 Teaspoon low-sodium margarine

Recipe Two

Easy Meal

- Ground turkey
- Bell peppers
- 1 Large pear or some cherries

Recipe Three

Easy Meal

- 1 Cup Rice Krispies cereals
- 1 Hard-boiled egg
- 1 Slice of white bread

Recipe Four

Beef and Broccoli Over Zucchini Noodles
Ingredients

- 1 Cup beef broth (without salt)
-1 Tablespoon corn starch
- 1Tablespoon lower-sodium soy sauce
- 2 Cloves garlic (minced)
- 1 Tablespoon fresh ginger (minced)
- 2 Tablespoons sesame oil (toasted)

- 1 Small onion
- 1 Lb sirloin beef (sliced)
- 4 Cups fresh broccoli florets
- 4 Cups zucchini noodles
- 2 Tablespoons sesame seeds
- 1 Nonstick cooking spray

Directions

1) Combine broth, cornstarch, soy sauce, ginger, and garlic in a small bowl and whisk until well mixed.

2) Spray a large sauté pan with cooking spray, pour in sesame oil, and then place on high heat.
3) Sauté onions for three minutes, then add in the beef and leave for another 3 -5 minutes.

4) Stir in zucchini and broccoli and stir fry for 3 minutes.

5) Slowly pour in the broth mixture, stirring so it doesn't form lumps.

6) Reduce the heat and leave to simmer for 5 minutes.

7) Add sesame oil and serve.

Other Food Options for a Diabetic CKD Individual

- Proteins: Unsalted seafood, eggs, poultry, and fish.

- Carbs: White bread, pasta, bagels, and sandwich buns
- Fruits: Berries, cherries, plums, grapes, pear, and peaches.

- Veggies: Turnips, eggplants, cauliflower, cucumber, broccoli, Lady's finger, cabbage, and onions.

Renal Diet Recipes for a Vegetarian

Recipe One

Maple Pancakes
Ingredients

- 1 Cup flour
- 2 Large egg whites
- 1 Cup low-fat milk (1%)
- 2 Tablespoons canola oil
- 1 Tablespoon granulated sugar
- 1 Tablespoon maple extract

- 2 Teaspoons baking powder
- ⅛ Teaspoon salt

Directions
1) Mix flour, salt, baking powder, and sugar in a large bowl. Create a hole in the center and set it aside.

2) In another bowl, mix maple extract, egg whites, milk, and oil, then pour into the first bowl.

3) Stir until both mixtures are well-mixed to create a slightly thick batter.

4) Lightly grease a skillet and place it on medium heat.

5) Pour a quarter cup batter into the pan and cook for 2 -3 minutes or until it turns a light golden brown before flipping over and doing the same for the other side.

Recipe Two

Pasta Primavera
Ingredients

- 10 Ounces pasta

- 10 Ounces mixed veggies (frozen)
- 12 Ounces low-sodium chicken broth
- 2 Tablespoons flour
- ½ Cup half and half
- ½ Cup Parmesan cheese (grated)
- ¼ Teaspoon garlic powder

Directions

1. Cook pasta without salt for five minutes and then Drain.

2. Cook broth in another pot, adding flour and whisking to keep it from forming lumps.

3. Stir in garlic powder and half and half then leave to simmer for 10 minutes.

4. Add cooked veggies and pasta and cook for another 3 -5 minutes.

5. Sprinkle Parmesan cheese and serve.

Chapter 9: Getting To Know Your Urinary Stones

One of the most agonizing and harrowing conditions that humans have to endure is a kidney stone attack. Kidney stones—scientifically called renal lithiasis—are not rare as 10-15% of adult Americans are victims of kidney stone at some time in their lives.

Each year, there are about 1 million Americans prone to kidney stones. Once you suffer from a single kidney stone attack, there is about 70-80% chance of its recurrence.

The risk of having kidney stones is traceable to family genetics. The younger you had your first attack; the higher will be your risk for a second one.

Kidney stones are not anything new as this was a known disorder even at the dawn of civilization. In fact, one of the earliest known surgical procedures is called Lithotomy, an operatic procedure for stone removal. In the Hippocratic Oath text, there is a warning about the risks of stones removal operation.

Sex-wise, the risk of kidney stones operation in the male is four times higher than in the female. Place-wise, the danger is greater for those living in U.S. southeastern area referred to as the "Kidney Stone Belt," because of dehydration.

Worldwide, kidney stone rates in the Middle East are nearly double than in the U.S., on account of the hotter climate.

It is interesting to know that kidney stones differ in sizes; the smallest are like grains of sand and the largest the size of a golf ball. If a stone is not removed, the urinary tract will be permanently damaged.

This condition should not be taken lightly as the about of a kidney stone attack is painful. Actually, VERY PAINFUL.

What is a kidney stone and how is it formed?

If you have seen a urinary stone, it is really a small solid formation of solidified minerals or salts in urine into crystals inside the kidney.

Soluble salts are substances in the kidney stones. Calcium oxalate is a kidney stone of the most common type developed from soluble salt either in a soluble form or as solid, crystalline.

In the process called precipitation, concentrated soluble salt is high enough so it begins to form into solid crystals. For instance, the common soluble salt called sodium chloride comes from seawater that is left to stand and evaporate. The precipitation coming out is the solution of sodium chloride in the form of sea-salt.

Urine has many chemical elements that form into soluble salts. The chemicals are usually found in a dissolved form in urine. However, salt concentrated in the urine are usually so much higher than could stay dissolved in pure water. This rare happening is due to the presence of urine inhibitors that make it more difficult to develop as soluble salt crystals.

Kidney stone inhibitors are sometimes substances found on a citrate diet while others are from proteins manufactured by human bodies that prevent the formation of stones. The body manufactures inhibitor proteins called Tamm-Horsfall protein and nephrocalcin.

The initial process in the formation of stones is known as nucleation. This takes place when there are factors encouraging salt crystals development is stronger than the factors inhibiting salt crystals to form. Following kidney stone are crystals getting larger over time and remains as such when urine conditions remain favorable for stone formation.

Some essential factors affecting the development of kidney stones are: (1) the amount of urine produced by the individual; (2) the lower volumes causing more concentration of urine; and (3) the slow condition of drainage that facilitates crystals to collect and combine.

It is easier for stones to begin constituting an anchor for crystals to develop on. "Randall's plaques "are kidney tissues that served as natural binding site where small calcifications can form.

Who is at risk of urinary stone formation?

Here are the risk factors of kidney stones:

Based on sex: men are more prone than women

Those with previous history of the disorder; at least 50% will come down with the stone within the next five years

Congenital: a family history of kidney stones

People between age 20 and 40

Dehydration - not drinking enough water

Improper diet high in protein

Those prescribed on certain meds such as diuretics /water tablets, antacids and drugs for thyroid

People with only a single kidney, or kidney that is abnormally shaped

What causes kidney stones?

In a rough estimate, a million Americans will develop kidney stones per year. In one's lifetime, about 10-15% of adults will develop kidney stone.

Even a single kidney stone attack is a risk as it has from 70 to 80% chance of recurring. The younger the sufferer of kidney stone, the more chances of its return.

The unwelcome kidney stone results when there is super-saturation of acid salts and minerals in the urine. Minerals like calcium and uric acid crystallize and form solid masses. This happens to people who do not have enough fluid intake and those with urine that is highly acidic or highly alkaline.

Even certain drugs promote the development of kidney stones, as Xenical, Lasix or furosemide, topomax or topiramate and some others. Contents of kidney stones are crystals of several types, with calcium plays the role of protagonist. However, there will be a single type of crystals predominating and determining the type that will be recognized as the basic.

Seventy-five percent of cases considered the most common type are the calcium oxalate stones. Oxalate is a chemical found in some fruits and veggies but it is the liver that produces most of the body's oxalate.

After analyzing the cause of stones, medical experts conclude that the best solution is to eliminate or seriously reduce calcium as its intake becomes part of the stone, but this is NOT a wise strategy.

Normally, the calcium in your diet is tied up to the oxalate, and it assists in the excretion of wastes other than urinating.

What are other types of stones and their underlying causes?

Struvite stones are more common in women as these stones are often in the unitary tract infection;

Uric acid stones are side effects of protein metabolism. Commonly accompanying gout; but the stones may be the effect of some genetic influences and blood-producing tissues' disorders;

A very small percentage of kidney stones are the Cystine that results from hereditary strains that cause the kidneys to emit a great deal amounts of certain amino acids or cystinuria.

Digestive problems and high blood pressure are two risky factors that elevate every man's chances of developing kidney stones.

Chapter 10: Dealing With Painful Kidney Stone Attack

A kidney stone attack is not only a serious condition but also a painful one.

Your kidneys are the organs responsible for removing excess fluid; at the same time, they filter out unneeded electrolytes and the wastes from the blood that produces urine.

When the minerals and acid salts in your urine solidify, kidney stones are formed when they stick together and form a solid mass. This results when the urine with more crystal-forming substances unites like calcium and uric acid is followed by the dilution of available fluid. This is also the result when urine is highly alkaline or highly acidic.

Kidney stones are also created when the kidney absorbs and eliminates calcium and other substances. Sometimes a kidney disease or a metabolic disorder is the underlying cause.

Xenical, Lasix or furosemide and topomax or topiramate are among the drugs promoting kidney stones. There are also many times factors combining in the environment that are favorable to stone formation.

Stones are not damaging until it is moved into the ureter that is the tube connecting the kidney and the bladder.

Common symptoms are:

Pain experienced along your side, back and below the ribs;

Incidence of pain lasting 20 to 60 minutes at varying intensity;

Radiating waves of pain traveling from side and back then to the lower abdomen and groin;

Foul-smelling urine that is cloudy containing blood;

Painful urination;

Episodes of nausea and vomiting;

Continuous urge to urinate; and

Fever and chills as indicators of infection.

Painful urination is due to the distention of the tissues over the stone as it blocks the passage of urine. It is not only due to the pressure of the stone itself.

Why is it painful?

The usual first cause of symptoms happens when the kidney stone tries to descend to the ureter and out of the urinary system. As it goes down the ureter, it causes blockage, leading to the development of increased pressure in the kidney above. It is this pressure that leads to the pain associated with passing a stone.

As it moves down the ureter, the stone tends to become lodged in three passages that are natural narrowing: (1) the crossing of the ureter above the iliac vessels; (2) the ureteropelvic junction; and (3) the entrance of the ureter into the bladder. Associated pain varies based on the location of stone along this path.

The pain follows a certain passage from high over near the kidney then travels towards the abdomen and goes down towards the groin as the stone goes further down the ureter. As the stone is emerging, patients have the urge to urinate.

What happens to immobile kidney stones?

Some doctors believe that kidney stones that are not blocking the ureter and are not trying to go down the bladder do not cause pain. Stones that are not obstructing as those located in the kidney's calyxes, are non-painful. This is the reason why some patients with extremely big stones in their entire kidney experienced no or at least only minimal pain.

In diagnosing kidney stones, doctors will collect samples and have them analyzed for a definitive answer, or make a 24-hour urine test. This is the best strategy to be sure of discovering any imbalances in that urine predisposes the growth of stones.

Chapter 11: Saying Goodbye To Kidney Stones

Another risk factor attributed to kidney stones is living a sedentary life. People who are bed-ridden or very inactive are more prone to kidney stones because immobility causes bones to release more calcium.

High blood pressure multiplies the risk of kidney stones.

Since changes in the digestive process affect calcium absorption, as well as other minerals, any problem of digestion increases the risk of stone kidney.

High-sugar diet high prioritizes stones, since sugar disrupts the mineral relationships in the body by obstructing the absorption of calcium and magnesium.

In addition, sugar and high fructose corn syrup cause obesity and diabetes, as well as the present trend in the over-consumption of unhealthy sugars by children. This is the factor why children as young as age 5 or 6 are developing kidney stones.

A South African study in 1999 concluded that drinking soda exacerbates a urine condition that forms calcium oxalate kidney stone problems.

Studies of diets high in processed salt are also bad news as salt increases calcium and oxalates in urine.

According to the report of co-director of pediatric urology at the University of Wisconsin Dr. Bruce L. Slaughenhoupt, a great increase in the salt load of children's diets from canned soups, French fries, sandwich meats and sports drinks like Gatorade, which are now sold in child-friendly juice boxes.

He believes that today most children over consume processed foods that cause increased kidney stones.

It is not a surprise that childhood obesity is linked to kidney stones. Children prefer drinking soda over water that adds to the problem.

Soy consumption develops kidney stones as it predisposes high levels of oxalate present in many varieties of soybeans. This is one more reason to junk non-fermented soy from your food itinerary.

And finally, caffeine is strongly linked to kidney stones. In an experiment, people with kidney stone history were given caffeine drinks and after their urine were examined. They showed high amount of urine calcium, placing them at a greater risk for kidney stones.

What of calcium intake?

Sufferers of kidney stones in the past were warned to keep away from foods rich in calcium. However, evidence emphasized that avoiding calcium is more harmful.

Studies conducted by the Harvard School of Public Health with more than 45,000 subjects revealed that those whose diets were rich in calcium had a one-third lower risk of kidney stones than those with lower calcium diets.

Why is this? After all, calcium is the largest component in the stones. The answer is that diet high in calcium actually impedes a chemical action that creates stones.

It ties up with oxalates from foods in the intestine that prevents both of them from being absorbed into the blood and later transferred to the kidneys. So it gives importance for urinary oxalates in the forming kidney stone calcium-oxalate crystals in comparison to urinary calcium.

It must be noted that calcium from foods is beneficial but not calcium supplements as they actually increase the risk of kidney stones by 20%.

Busting the Myth That High Protein Diets Led To Kidney Stones

Diet advocates will recall that when the 1990 Atkins diet was enormously popular, critics claimed that high protein causes kidney stones. This is both a myth and misinformation.

People suffering from kidney disease are given protein restricted diet; however, eating meat is not the cause of kidney problem. In fact, the fat-soluble vitamins and saturated fat in animal meats play a great role in proper functioning of the kidneys.

More On What To Do And Not To Do For Healthier Kidneys

Aside from being the safest and simplest in handling stones, the best approach is allowing the stones to pass on their own. No need to consider time as the process might take days, or weeks in several cases but the key is to drink enough water (not soda) to decrease solid concentration in the urine until the stone is dissolved.

If coffee is a no – no, so is tea since it is rich in oxalates.

Several medical procedures and surgical techniques are used to remedy kidney stones, but there is high risk that physicians use the remedy as the last resort. This practice is actually beneficial as many American patients are facing problems due to medical errors.

Pain relievers are the best methods to relieve intolerable pain.

Some medicinal herbs have been very helpful in handling acute episodes, these include:

Bearberry

Cleavers

Corn Silk

Crampbark
Gravel Root
Hydrangea
Kava Kava
Khella
Hydrangea
Nettle Leaf
Stone Root

For the most effective use of herbs, get the advice of an expert herbalist as herbs can be every bit a very potent pharmaceutical product and maybe harmful if improperly used.

If you have been living a healthy life and had allowed the natural passage of kidney stones, you would not have to deal with this very painful problem in the first place.

Modifying Your Lifestyle For Healthier Kidneys

Just a few changes in your lifestyle will go a long way in preventing painful kidney stone attack.

Always stay well- hydrated

Adopt a diet based on the unique nutritional type of your body;

Remember that taking prescription drugs cause more harm than healing;

Caffeine, excess salt, soy, sugar and processed foods are out of your menu;

Keep body fluid on the go by plenty of exercise;

Include in your diet adequate amount of Vitamin B6 and magnesium as they are great in blocking formation of kidney stone.

Changing one's lifestyle is always tedious and requires many efforts. At first, it is inconvenient but you have to remember passing a kidney stone is a painful process so a few lifestyle changes will not look dismal.

Do not force yourself to adopt a diet or start an exercise routine.

Be eager to adopt a healthy lifestyle and everything else will fall into place. With healthy choices and healthy things to do while keeping your mind and body positive, dieting and exercising are cinch.

By motivating your mind to live healthy and surrounding yourself with healthy things; you will find renewed energy. It will no longer require efforts to shed a few pounds, no efforts to look great, no prompting to feel health and no motivation to stay that way. Do it as a gift to yourself, your family and your kids.

Through proper healthy diet, you rid your body of kidney stones and prevent them from forming. Proper diet does not mean sacrificing your palate, you can combine fresh fruits and veggies that are delicious and learn to cook appetizing meals.

Processed frozen food may be the best choice for people who simply do not have the time for home cooked meals. But there is no doubt that cooked meals made from fresh ingredients are so much healthier.

It is also a good idea to give up sugary sodas; water is free and an essential part of what your body needs.

You have to exercise regularly so the bones absorb calcium coming from the blood that prevents it from forming in the kidneys. Set an exercise schedule full of different activities; you can choose from: aerobics, bicycling, boxing, dancing, videos exercise, weight training, yoga, pilates, stair climbing and many more.

You will not get bored when your activities are varied. Changing scheduled exercise routine will make the task of staying fit an interesting aspect of your daily activities. A weekly shopping or daily walk to your office can be an added incentive in your physical activity.

Choose to climb a few flights of stairs instead of using the escalator or the elevator. Instead of riding lawnmower, you can push one around the yard. Use the chores around the house as a leeway to keep fit.

Everything you do is an added bonus to stay fit. Dancing in time to the radio can blow off a little steam, jump on your bed or stay in motion to lose weight, just keep moving.

Flushing Out Toxins From Your System

Water and water is the best way to flush out your system. It would go a long way towards preventing kidney stone as well as flushing them out by drinking from 6 to 8, eight ounce glasses of water a day. Increase your fluid intake to help ward off kidney stones by adding broths, juices and soups to your diet.

An increase your fluid intake is needed because the natural production of kidney fluid is only one liter. If the kidney urine is concentrated, then minerals would crystallize and kidney stones are formed. So by drinking lots of fluids, it flushes out your kidneys and keeps them healthy.

The Vitamins You Shouldn't Be Without

Tip Number One - Vitamin supplements increases kidney stones so get your vita- min intake from foods.

Vitamin A is great for your diet. Roughage foods are fiber-rich as legumes, grains, nuts, seeds and others promote healthy kidney. You can incorporate in your daily meal two servings of food rich in Vit. A.

Vitamin B6 is good for your kidneys. Try to incorporate at least 2 servings of the foods rich in these vitamins in your daily diet.

Magnesium provides more than 300 biochemical reactions in your body. Magnesium has been linked to kidney stones for it is a protagonist in the body's absorption and assimilation of calcium.

The problem is that if the body takes in too much calcium without the adequate amount of magnesium, the excess amount of calcium turns toxic and contributes to the growth of kidney stones.

Magnesium helps to keep calcium from joining with oxalate that is the most common type of kidney stone.

Excellent source of magnesium are green leafy veggies like Swiss chard and spinach. One way to ascertain that you are consuming enough amount of magnesium is of by juicing your vegetables. Juices squeezed from vegetables are teeming with magnesium.

Also consider nuts as almonds, beans, seeds from pumpkin, sunflower and sesame. Avocadoes are delicious and also a good source. However, surveys shows that despite the abundance of food, many Americans do not contain enough magnesium in their diets.

According to Carolyn Dean, MD, ND, who authored The Miracle of Magnesium, there is an estimate of more than 80% of population in America deficient in magnesium.

To use magnesium as supplement, it is important to understand that it is a partner complementary to calcium. So have to use both. You can even double elemental dose of magnesium relative to the elemental calcium. The ratio works out quite fine for both.

These Things Should Be Reduced

Protein

The daily recommendation of protein intake is 50 grams; however, proteins from animal contain purines that increase the formation of calcium, phosphorus and uric acid in the urine that forms painful stones in the kidneys.

There are other sources of protein from chicken and plants. You can get protein from lean cuts of chicken as it is rich in vitamin B6 that fights off the formation of oxalates in the body.

Incorporate at least 3 ounces of chicken into your diet daily. For more, get from plants such as:

Almonds

Cashews

Peas

Lentils

Grains

Soy

Tofu

Vitamin C

Reduce your intake of vitamin C for so much of this vitamin increases your chance of having kidney stones. Keep away from Vitamin C Supplements as the best source of Vitamin C comes naturally from food. It is allowable to take Vitamin C enriched foods but limited to one serving per day.

These are rich in Vitamin C:

Brussels Sprouts

Cantaloupe

Green or Red Pepper

Guava

Kiwi

Oranges

Eliminate These From Your Diet

No to Oxalates – Oxalate makes up kidney stones so avoid as it binds with calcium and causes painful kidney stone.

No to Sugar, fructose and soda –A diet high in sugar is the best way to court kidney stones, as sugar agitates the mineral relationships of the body by obstructing the absorption of calcium and magnesium.

Children's consumption of unhealthy sodas and sugars is a large factor why kinds as young as five or six are already developing kidney stones. One South African research concluded that drinking soda heightens conditions in your urine that leading to the formation of calcium oxalate kidney stone problems. Sugar is detrimental as it increases the size of kidney and produces pathological changes as the formation of kidney stones.

No to Grapefruit Juice – Although most juices are safe but grapefruit juice is not and is discovered to be an increased risk of kidney stones. So it is best to stay away from it.

No to Salt/Sodium – Consumption of sodium increases calcium in the urine that is the major factor in developing painful kidney stones. Sodium includes salt. Sodium is found heavily in packaged and processed foods. Be alert of high sodium content in breads, canned foods, cheeses, soft drinks and frozen foods.

No to these Purines – it is best to eliminate food containing purines such as alcoholic beverages, asparagus, beans, beets. blackberries, bread, canned soups, canned veggies, celery, cheeses, chocolates, draft beers, eggplants, frozen dinners, herring, mackerels, mussels, organ meats, parsley, peanuts, rhubarbs, sardines, soft drinks, soy products, strawberries, string beans, sweet potatoes and yeast.

Remedy #1: Apples

This is true to the statement that an apple a day drives kidney stones away. Include an apple in your daily diet to prevent formation of kidney stones from uric acid.

Remedy #2: Celery

These veggies are one of the most potent ingredients in dealing with kidney stones. Include celery in your daily meal to maintain a health kidney.

Remedy #3: Coconut Water

A regular intake of coco water will go a long way in preventing formation of kidney stones. Coconut water also works great in breaking down kidney stones and helps in facilitating their passage through the urinary tract.

Remedy #4: Kidney Beans

Soak kidney beans in a bowl of water overnight. Then cut them and add to four liters of boiling water turn on low and boil for 8 hours. Remove from heat to cool. Strain the liquid and a glass of the kidney bean juice every two hours for the first day. Then drink one glass every for the following few days. Kidney bean juice reduces the size of uric acid stones so they easily pass through the system.

Remedy # 5: Lemons

Lemons are great in helping cleanse your kidneys and preventing kidney stones from forming. Lemons contain citrate, which is nature's inhibitor of the formation of kidney stone and lemons contain the highest concentration of citrate than any other fruit.

Lemons can be done two ways:

1. Drink lemon juice – Mix four ounces of lemon juice and two liters of water and drink daily. This beverage will decrease the chance of kidney stones formation; and

2. Drink a combo of lemon juice and olive oil – Mix four ounces of lemon juice and two ounces of olive oil. Wash it down with a large glass of water. This remedy caused kidney stones to pass within a 24 hour period.

Remedy #6: Onions

Although the taste may not be to your liking but this is very effective. Cook 2 medium-sized onions and 2 cups f water over medium flame. Remove from heat and allow to cool. Place the concoction in a blender. Drink one glass of the juice for 3 days to eliminate kidney stone from your system.

Remedy #7: Good Orange Juice

With oranges, you can never go wrong. Drink one glass of orange juice once a day and this is the best option to prevent kidney stones much better than other fruits.

Chapter 12: What Exactly Is Kidney Failure?

Your kidneys can lose up to 90% of their function while still performing admirably. If you lose more than that, you have renal failure.

Kidney failure is classified into two types:

Acute renal failure is characterized by a sudden decrease in kidney function. It is typically reversible.

Chronic renal failure is characterized by a progressive loss of kidney function. It worsens over time and is irreversible (but you can slow its progression).

When your kidneys fail, waste and extra fluid accumulate in your body. This results in renal failure symptoms.

What is the root cause of kidney failure?
Acute renal failure happens when your kidneys are abruptly unable to function as a result of an external cause. Some of the contributing factors are as follows:

acute pyelonephritis is a type of kidney infection (kidney infection) substantial blood loss as a result of dehydration

extremely low blood pressure

In some imaging procedures, such as CT or MRI scans, a special dye is employed.

glomerulonephritis is a type of kidney disease (damage to the filtering parts of your kidney) NSAIDs (nonsteroidal anti-inflammatory drugs) over-the-counter pain relievers (NSAIDs) prescribed medications (including some blood pressure medications at high doses, antibiotics, or cancer treatments) other medications (such as heroin, cocaine, and amphetamines) other medications (such as heroin, cocaine, and amphetamines)

Chronic kidney failure happens when something affects your kidneys over time and a long period. The following are some of the reasons:

Diabetes is associated with high blood pressure.

It can be caused by hereditary disorders, such as polycystic kidney disease, or by glomerulonephritis that is slow and progressive. It can also be caused by slow and progressive interstitial nephritis.

kidney infection caused by autoimmune illnesses such as lupus nephritis and Goodpasture syndrome, which can be chronic or recurrent

Kidney Failure Symptoms
In the early stages of renal failure, there are usually no symptoms. When they do arise, the following symptoms may occur:

confusion

decreased urine flow, weariness, problems concentrating, itching, muscular twitching, and a metallic taste in your mouth

vomiting and nausea

Seizures due to loss of appetite

Edema (body swelling) that begins in the ankles and legs (peripheral edema)

shortness of breath caused by an accumulation of fluid in your lungs

a defect (asthenia)

What are the consequences of renal failure?
Aside from filtering your blood, your kidneys perform a variety of additional functions. When the kidneys fail, they are unable to perform these functions, and problems may arise.

anemia

coronary heart disease

blood pressure is too high

hyperkalemia is a condition in which the body's (high potassium levels in your blood)

Pericarditis is an infection of the heart (inflammation of the lining around your heart)

malnutrition

osteoporosis is a disease that causes bone loss (weak bones)

neuropathy of the extremities (nerve damage in your legs)

a weakened immune system

11 ways to prevent kidney failure
Because high blood pressure and diabetes are the two most common causes of kidney failure, many of the prevention tips revolve around controlling these two illnesses.

1. Maintain a healthy blood sugar level.

Diabetes increases your chances of developing heart disease and renal failure. That is only one reason to keep your blood sugar under control.

2. Maintain a healthy blood pressure level

High blood pressure might put you at risk for heart disease and renal failure.

3. Keep a healthy weight

Obesity can increase your risk of renal failure-related illnesses such as diabetes and high blood pressure.

4. Consume a heart-healthy diet
A heart-healthy diet is low in sugar and cholesterol while being high in fiber, whole grains, and fruits and vegetables.

5. Limit your salt consumption.

Excessive salt consumption is linked to high blood pressure.

6. Drink plenty of water

Dehydration lowers blood flow to the kidneys, which can be harmful. Consult your doctor about how much water you should drink each day.

7. Keep alcohol to a minimum

Your blood pressure rises when you consume alcohol. The extra calories in it can also cause you to gain weight.

8. Don't smoke.

Cigarette smoking lowers blood flow to the kidneys. It impairs renal function in those who have or do not have kidney disease.
9. Limit your use of over-the-counter pain relievers.

Nonsteroidal anti-inflammatory medicines (NSAIDs) such as aspirin, ibuprofen, and naproxen, in high doses, restrict blood flow to your kidneys, which might injure them.

10. Lessen your stress

Reducing stress and worry can help lower blood pressure, which is beneficial to your kidneys.

11. Exercise regularly

Swimming, walking, and jogging are all forms of exercise that can help you reduce stress, manage diabetes and high blood pressure, and maintain a healthy weight.

If you suspect you have kidney illness, make an appointment with your doctor very away. Getting a diagnosis and therapy as soon as possible will help reduce the progression to renal failure.

If you know you have kidney disease, see your doctor regularly to have your kidney function checked. While chronic kidney disease cannot be reversed, it can be slowed with the right treatment.

Is there a way to treat kidney failure?
Both types of renal failure can be treated. Acute renal failure is reversible. The progression of

chronic kidney failure can be delayed with the correct medication.

The difficulty is only transient in acute renal failure. Once the problem is resolved, your kidneys will resume normal function. Treatment examples include:

antibiotics for pyelonephritis blood transfusion

Immune disorders are treated with corticosteroids.

Dehydration is treated with intravenous fluids.

removing an impediment

If your kidneys do not respond to treatment straight away, hemodialysis might be used to keep them working until they do.

Chronic renal failure is caused by progressive kidney injury. Because it is irreversible, something else must take over the task of your kidneys. The alternatives are as follows:

Hemodialysis. Your blood can be filtered by a dialysis machine. This can be done at a dialysis center or home, but you will need a partner.

Peritoneal dialysis is a type of kidney dialysis. The filtration takes place in your abdomen. This can be done in a facility or at home. It does not necessitate the assistance of a spouse.

Transplantation of a kidney A transplanted kidney is surgically implanted into your body.

What to anticipate if you are diagnosed with kidney failure

Your prognosis is determined by the type of renal failure.

If you have chronic kidney failure, your kidneys will not heal, but you can delay the progression of the disease with the correct treatment unless you receive a kidney transplant.

If you suffer acute renal failure, your kidneys will almost certainly heal and begin to function again.

The main point

Following these guidelines can help you avoid or delay the course of renal failure. The most important thing you can do is keep your diabetes and high blood pressure under control.

Another important factor in maintaining your kidneys healthy is to have a healthy lifestyle that includes eating well, staying active, and not smoking.

Natural Herbs for Improved Kidney Function
Tea made from dandelion flowers.

The root of the marshmallow

Juniper.

Nettles.

Parsley.

The red clover.

Ginger.

Goldenrod.
Home-based complementary therapies
Some people opt to treat medical ailments using natural or alternative treatments.

Because kidney infections are so dangerous, you mustn't rely on home cures. Instead, take the medicines prescribed by your doctor and employ home remedies to alleviate symptoms or pain. Home treatments can also be used to prevent UTIs and enhance kidney function.

1. Consume plenty of water

Drinking enough water can assist in flushing bacteria from the body, allowing the infection to be cleared more quickly. It can also aid in the elimination of toxins from the urinary tract.

Drinking plenty of water can also help to prevent UTIs, which can lead to kidney infections, so it's a smart habit to maintain. Aim for at least eight glasses of fluids per day.

2. Consume cranberry juice
Cranberry juice has long been used to treat urinary tract infections and bladder infections. Some data suggest that consuming cranberry juice may help or prevent UTIs in some persons.

Many individuals prefer cranberry juice to water because it has a sweeter flavor, which encourages them to drink more. Cranberry juices with additional sweets, on the other hand, are not good for you. A cranberry supplement or pure cranberry juice is a healthier method to reap cranberry advantages.

3. Avoid alcoholic beverages and coffee.

The kidneys' most crucial function is to filter out dangerous substances and poisons, and both alcohol and caffeine can cause the kidneys to work overtime. This may impede the healing process after an infection. Alcohol and antibiotics should not be combined, therefore avoid alcohol during your therapy for the same reason.

4. Consume probiotics

When it comes to treating kidney infections, probiotics have two major advantages. The first is that they will assist keep your body's beneficial bacteria in balance, even though antibiotics may kill both "good" and "bad" bacteria.

There is also evidence that probiotics can help the kidneys process waste, and the better your kidneys function, the more effective your treatment will be.

5. Consume some vitamin C

Vitamin C is a potent antioxidant that protects tissues in the body from oxidative stress, hence promoting kidney function. There is also previous evidence that demonstrates vitamin C can decrease kidney scarring after acute renal infection and enhance enzymes within the kidneys. You can get vitamin C from supplements or meals high in the substance.

6. Make use of parsley juice

Parsley juice is a nutrient-dense diureticTrusted Source that can increase urine frequency and volume. This can help wash out bacteria in the kidneys more quickly, making antibiotics more effective. If you don't like the taste of parsley, combine it with strong-flavored fruits such as cranberries or blueberries for the best results.

7. Eat apples and apple juice

Apples are also high in nutrients. Their high acid content may aid the kidneys in maintaining urine acidity, thereby limiting future bacterial growth. They also have anti-inflammatory qualities, which may aid in the healing of the kidneys after infection. Find out more about the numerous health benefits of apples.

8. Take a bath with Epsom salts.

Epsom salts and warm water can also help to relieve discomfort. This can help to make the unpleasant side effects of the kidney infection more bearable while you wait for the antibiotics to kick in.

Because abdominal pain can be a symptom of both antibiotics and kidney infections, this could be beneficial even after the symptoms of the kidney infection have subsided. Learn how to make an Epsom salt detox bath as well as any side effects to be aware of.

9. Use pain medicines that do not contain aspirin.

Non-aspirin pain medications can be effective in relieving discomfort. Ibuprofen (Motrin and Advil) and acetaminophen (Tylenol) can also help break fevers produced by the virus.

10. Use heat

Heat therapy might help relieve discomfort while you wait for the antibiotics to take effect. Apply a heating pad or a hot water bottle to the affected area for about 20 minutes at a time.

Chapter 13: Kidneys & How They Work

The kidneys are two bean-shaped organs, each about the size of a fist. They are located just below the rib cage, one on each side of your spine.

Healthy kidneys filter about a half cup of blood every minute, removing wastes and extra water to make urine. The urine flows from the kidneys to the bladder through two thin tubes of muscle called ureters, one on each side of your bladder. Your bladder stores urine. Your kidneys, ureters, and bladder are part of your urinary tract. You have two kidneys that filter your blood, removing wastes and extra water to make urine.

Renal function

Kidney function or renal function depends on the efficiency of the kidneys to filter the blood and is estimated using glomerular filtration rate (GFR). The amount of filtrate that forms every minute (min) within the glomerulus is called the GFR. A person"s estimated GFR (eGFR) is the best indicator of how well the kidneys are functioning.

In adults, the GFR is approximately 120 mL/min. Gradual loss of kidney function is called chronic kidney disease (CKD). A person with GFR less than 60 mL/min per $1.73m2$ of body surface area for three months or longer is classified as having CKD, irrespective of the presence or absence of kidney damage. Kidney damage is defined as pathologic abnormalities or markers of damage, including abnormalities in blood or urine test or imaging studies. All individuals with kidney damage are classified as having CKD, irrespective of the level of GFR. Risk factors for CKD include diabetes, high blood pressure, family history, older age, ethnic group and smoking. Evaluation methods for people at increased risk of CKD are to measure urine albumin and red blood cells in the urine to assess kidney damage and to estimate the GFR with an equation based on the level of serum creatinine. GFR of 90 or above is considered normal. The severity of CKD is described by five stages:

1) Stage 1 – Slightly diminished function; kidney damage with normal or relatively high GFR (above 90)

2) Stage 2 – Mild reduction in GFR of 60 to 89 with kidney damage

3) Stage 3 – Moderate reduction in GFR of 30 to 59

4) Stage 4 – Severe reduction in GFR of 15 to 29

5) Stage 5 – Established kidney failure with GFR of less than 15

Total and permanent kidney failure is called end stage renal disease (ESRD). People with ESRD must undergo dialysis or kidney transplantation for treating last stages of kidney failure.

Dialysis is the artificial process used to maintain the chemical composition of the blood. Hemodialysis (HD) and peritoneal dialysis are the two major forms of dialysis.

HD uses a cellulose membrane tube or filter called a dialyzer that functions as an artificial kidney to clean a person's blood. Peritoneal dialysis uses the lining of the patient's abdominal cavity, known as the peritoneum as the dialysis membrane to clean a person's blood. Kidney transplantation involves replacing a patient's failed kidney with a kidney from a healthy donor.

Chronic kidney disease: the global challenge

The worldwide rise in the number of patients with CKD"s is reflected in the increasing number of people with ESRD treated by renal replacement therapy (RRT)- dialysis or transplantation. The health burden of renal disease is high for patients and health services worldwide. In Australia, approximately sixteen percent of the population have some form of kidney damage present and are therefore at risk of renal disease. Every year in Australia, almost one percent of adults developed CKD and another one percent of adults developed evidence of kidney damage. The rate of people with a kidney transplant or receiving dialysis in Australia rose by twenty six percent between 2006 and 2007. CKD contributed to nearly ten percent of all deaths in 2006 and over a million Australian dollars (AUD) hospitalisations in the year 2006- 2007 in Australia. Indigenous Australians were six times as likely as other Australians to be receiving dialysis or to have had a kidney transplant. Australia"s annual spending on end stage kidney disease (ESKD) is at least five hundred and seventy million dollars (AUD), and this is increasing annually by thirty million AUD. By 2012, the cost of maintaining people on hemodialysis will be thirty billion United States dollars (USD) for the United States (US) and eleven hundred billion USD worldwide.

More than fifteen percent of people in the US of age twenty or older have CKD. In the United Kingdom (UK), analysis of prevalent transplants by CKD showed fifteen percent. The overall incidence rate of RRT for ESRD across Europe in 2007 was hundred and sixteen per million population (pmp). CKD is more prevalent in Africa and seems to be of a more severe form than is found in Western countries. No reliable statistics describe CKD in all African countries, India and Pakistan. The majority of those with CKD die because of lack of funds, as very few can afford regular maintenance dialysis in Africa. Due to the cost constraints, only about five percent of all patients with CKD in India and Pakistan end up having a transplant. Nephrologic work in China started in early nineteen sixty"s. Approximately five thousand patients receive renal transplantation every year. The incidence of ESRD in China is estimated to be hundred and two pmp.

TRADITIONAL MEDICINE

World health organisation (WHO) defines TM as including diverse health practices, approaches, knowledge and beliefs incorporating plant, animal, and/or mineral based medicines, spiritual therapies, manual techniᐧues and exercises applied singularly or in combination to maintain well-being, as well as to treat, diagnose or prevent illness.

TM refers to TM systems such as TCM, Indian ayurveda and Arabic unani medicine. A variety of indigenous systems have also been developed throughout history by Asian, African, Arabic, Native American, Oceanic, Central and South American and other cultures. The term complementary and alternative medicine (CAM) is used instead of TM in countries like Europe and/or North America and Australia to refer to a broad set of health care practices that are not part of a country"s own tradition, or not integrated into its dominant health care system.

Widespread and growing use of traditional medicine
TM is widely used and is a rapidly growing health system of economic importance. In Africa up to eighty percent of the population uses TM to help meet their health care needs. In China, TM accounts for around forty percent of all health care delivered, and is used to treat roughly two hundred million patients annually. For Latin America, the WHO Regional Office for the Americas reported that seventy one percent of the population in Chile and forty percent of the population in Colombia have used TM. The percentage of the population that have used CAM at least once is forty two percent in United States of America (USA), forty nine percent in France, seventy percent in Canada and forty eight percent in Australia. In UK, almost forty percent of all general allopathic practitioners offer some form of CAM referral or access.

Expenditure of traditional medicine

In many parts of the world expenditure on TM/CAM is not only significant, but growing rapidly. Annual revenues in Western Europe reached five billion USD in 2003-2004. In China sales of products totalled fourteen billion USD in 2005. Herbal medicine revenue in Brazil was one hundred and sixty million USD in 2007. In Malaysia, an estimated five hundred million USD is spent annually on TM/CAM, compared to about three hundred million USD on allopathic medicine. In Australia, an estimated annual national expenditure on CAM and CAM practitioners is almost one thousand million AUD. Of this, six hundred and twenty one million AUD is spent on alternative medicines. A study of the practice of TCM in Australia, commissioned by the Victorian Department of Human services, New South Wales Department of Health, and the Queensland Department of Health, showed that the popularity of TCM was growing strongly. It is estimated that there are at least three million AUD TCM consultations each year in Australia. This represents an annual turnover of eighty four million AUD. The increasing popularity of TCM is also reflected in the four-fold increase in imports of Chinese herbal medicine (CHM) since 1992. In US, Canada and the UK, an annual CAM expenditure is estimated at twenty seven hundred million

USD, twenty four hundred million USD and twenty three hundred million USD respectively. The world market for herbal medicines based on traditional knowledge is now estimated at sixty thousand million USD.

Why are the kidneys important?

Your kidneys remove wastes and extra fluid from your body. Your kidneys also remove acid that is produced by the cells of your body and maintain a healthy balance of water, salts, and minerals—such as sodium, calcium, phosphorus, and potassium—in your blood.

Without this balance, nerves, muscles, and other tissues in your body may not work normally.

Your kidneys also make hormones that help
• control your blood pressure
• make red blood cells NIH external link
• keep your bones strong and healthy

How do my kidneys work?

Each of your kidneys is made up of about a million filtering units called nephrons. Each nephron includes a filter, called the glomerulus, and a tubule. The nephrons work through a two-step process: the glomerulus filters your blood, and the tubule returns needed substances to your blood and removes wastes.

Each nephron has a glomerulus to filter your blood and a tubule that returns needed substances to your blood and pulls out additional wastes. Wastes and extra water become urine.

The glomerulus filters your blood
As blood flows into each nephron, it enters a cluster of tiny blood vessels—the glomerulus. The thin walls of the glomerulus allow smaller molecules, wastes, and fluid—mostly water—to pass into the tubule. Larger molecules, such as proteins and blood cells, stay in the blood vessel.

The tubule returns needed substances to your blood and removes wastes
A blood vessel runs alongside the tubule. As the filtered fluid moves along the tubule, the blood vessel reabsorbs almost all of the water, along with minerals and nutrients your body needs. The tubule helps remove excess acid from the blood. The remaining fluid and wastes in the tubule become urine.

How does blood flow through my kidneys?
Blood flows into your kidney through the renal artery. This large blood vessel branches into smaller and smaller blood vessels until the

blood reaches the nephrons. In the nephron, your blood is filtered by the tiny blood vessels of the glomeruli and then flows out of your kidney through the renal vein.

Your blood circulates through your kidneys many times a day. In a single day, your kidneys filter about 150 quarts of blood. Most of the water and other substances that filter through your glomeruli are returned to your blood by the tubules. Only 1 to 2 quarts become urine.

Blood flows into your kidneys through the renal artery and exits through the renal vein. Your ureter carries urine from the kidney to your bladder.

 Function

The kidneys filter extra water and toxins from the blood. The kidneys filter about 120 to 152 quarts (113 to 144 liters) of blood to create 1 to 2 quarts (0.94 to 1.8 l) of urine every day, according to the National Institutes of Health (NIH).

They aren't just one big filtering sponge, though. Each kidney is a system of millions of tiny filters called nephrons. A nephron has two parts. The glomerulus is the first part of the filter. It strains blood cells and large molecules from the toxins and fluid. The fluids and toxins that pass through then go through the tubule.

The tubule collects minerals that the body needs and puts them back into the bloodstream and filters out more toxins.

While filtering, the kidneys produce urine to carry the toxins away. The urine is sent through two tubes called ureters down to the bladder, where the urine then leaves the body through the urethra.

The kidneys also make hormones. These hormones help regulate blood pressure, make red blood cells and promote bone health.

Conditions

Poor kidney care and genetics can cause a wide range of health problems. Chronic kidney disease, also called chronic kidney failure, is when the kidneys slowly stop functioning. One in three American adults are at high risk for developing kidney disease, according to the National Kidney Foundation. There are many conditions that can cause kidney disease, including type 1 and 2 diabetes, high blood pressure, obstructions in the urinary tract and inflammation of various parts of the kidneys, according to the Mayo Clinic.

Kidney failure is the most severe stage of kidney disease. It occurs when kidneys stop functioning without help. People with kidney failure need dialysis or a kidney transplant to survive. People with healthy kidneys can donate part of a kidney or a whole kidney to those in need without becoming sick, in most cases. Kidney transplants are one of the most common surgeries in the United States, according to the U.S. National Library of Medicine.

Kidney cancer is the seventh most common type of cancer. According to the Mayo Clinic, the most common type of kidney cancer is renal cell carcinoma. In the United States, 61,560 adults will be diagnosed with kidney cancer and renal pelvic cancer in 2015, and it will be the cause of around 14,080 deaths in 2015, according to the American Society of Clinical Oncology.

Kidney stones are exactly what they sound like. They are stones made from hardened minerals and acid salts that collect in the kidneys, usually formed by concentrated urine. The minerals in the urine crystalize and stick together, according to the Mayo Clinic. Though they are very painful, they usually don't cause any damage to the body.

Kidney infections, also called pyelonephritis, are usually caused by bacteria that enter the urethra, ascend into the bladder and make their way to the kidneys, according to the Urology Care Foundation. If a kidney infection goes untreated, it can cause permanent kidney damage.

Promoting good kidney health
Proper care can keep kidneys running properly well into old age. One of the most important things to remember is to stay hydrated. Kidneys need water to function properly and to carry away toxins.

"In the most serious cases, dehydration can eventually harm the body causing seizures, kidney failure and even death," said Dr. Buck Parker, a trauma surgeon who also recently appeared on NBC's reality TV show "The Island." Parker suggested that the best ways to avoid dehydration included drinking water before you get thirsty, since thirst indicates dehydration; eating foods, like fruits and vegetables, with a high water content; avoiding soda or other caffeinated drinks; and limiting alcohol consumption.

Vitamins can be very important to the function and health of kidneys. "(Folic acid) helps to reduce levels of homocysteine, which has been linked to heart disease, stroke and kidney disease," said Dr. Kristine Arthur, an internist at Orange Coast Memorial Medical Center in Fountain Valley, California. Vitamin A is also very important to healthy kidney function.

Taking too much vitamin C, though, may lead to kidney stones, according to Arthur.

Another supplement that may cause trouble is calcium. "Some older women who get their calcium from supplements rather than in their diet are more prone to kidney stones," said Dr. Linda Girgis, a family practice doctor in South River, New Jersey. "Many people falsely assume that taking vitamins is healthy and safe, but this is not always the case. Sometimes people take too much. It is very hard to get too much when ingesting it is food," said Girgis.

Keeping blood pressure in check may also contribute to long-term good kidney health. A study by the National Kidney Foundation found that moderately high blood pressure levels in midlife might contribute to late-life kidney disease and kidney failure.

The American Kidney Fund also suggests avoiding a diet high in fat and salt, limiting alcohol, avoiding tobacco and exercising most days as good ways to keep kidneys healthy.

What is kidney disease?

The kidneys are a pair of fist-sized organs located at the bottom of the rib cage. There is one kidney on each side of the spine.

Kidneys are essential to having a healthy body. They are mainly responsible for filtering waste products, excess water, and other impurities out of the blood. These toxins are stored in the bladder and then removed during urination. The kidneys also regulate pH, salt, and potassium levels in the body. They produce hormones that regulate blood pressure and control the production of red blood cells. The kidneys even activate a form of vitamin D that helps the body absorb calcium.

Kidney disease affects approximately 26 million American adults. It occurs when your kidneys become damaged and can't perform their function. Damage may be caused by diabetes, high blood pressure, and various other chronic (long-term) conditions. Kidney disease can lead to other health problems, including weak bones, nerve damage, and malnutrition.

If the disease gets worse over time, your kidneys may stop working completely. This means that dialysis will be required to perform the function of the kidneys. Dialysis is a treatment that filters and purifies the blood using a machine. It can't cure kidney disease, but it can prolong your life.

Chronic kidney disease

The most common form of kidney disease is chronic kidney disease. Chronic kidney disease is a long-term condition that doesn't improve over time. It's commonly caused by high blood pressure.

High blood pressure is dangerous for the kidneys because it can increase the pressure on the glomeruli. Glomeruli are the tiny blood vessels in the kidneys where blood is cleaned. Over time, the increased pressure damages these vessels and kidney function begins to decline.

Kidney function will eventually deteriorate to the point where the kidneys can no longer perform their job properly. In this case, a person would need to go on dialysis. Dialysis filters extra fluid and waste out of the blood. Dialysis can help treat kidney disease but it can't cure it. A kidney transplant may be another treatment option depending on your circumstances.

Diabetes is also a major cause of chronic kidney disease. Diabetes is a group of diseases that causes high blood sugar. The increased level of sugar in the blood damages the blood vessels in the kidneys over time. This means the kidneys can't clean the blood properly. Kidney failure can occur when your body becomes overloaded with toxins.

Kidney stones

Kidney stones are another common kidney problem. They occur when minerals and other substances in the blood crystallize in the kidneys, forming solid masses (stones). Kidney stones usually come out of the body during urination. Passing kidney stones can be extremely painful, but they rarely cause significant problems.

Glomerulonephritis
Glomerulonephritis is an inflammation of the glomeruli. Glomeruli are extremely small structures inside the kidneys that filter the blood. Glomerulonephritis can be caused by infections, drugs, or congenital abnormalities (disorders that occur during or shortly after birth). It often gets better on its own.

Polycystic kidney disease
Polycystic kidney disease is a genetic disorder that causes numerous cysts (small sacs of fluid) to grow in the kidneys. These cysts can interfere with kidney function and cause kidney failure. (It's important to note that individual kidney cysts are fairly common and almost always harmless. Polycystic kidney disease is a separate, more serious condition.)

Urinary tract infections
Urinary tract infections (UTIs) are bacterial infections of any part of the urinary system.

Infections in the bladder and urethra are the most common. They are easily treatable and rarely lead to more health problems. However, if left untreated, these infections can spread to the kidneys and cause kidney failure.

What are the symptoms of kidney disease?
Kidney disease is a condition that can easily go unnoticed until the symptoms become severe. The following symptoms are early warning signs that you might be developing kidney disease:
• fatigue
• difficulty concentrating
• trouble sleeping
• poor appetite
• muscle cramping
• swollen feet/ankles
• puffiness around the eyes in the morning
• dry, scaly skin
• freᐧuent urination, especially late at night
Severe symptoms that could mean your kidney disease is progressing into kidney failure include:
• nausea
• vomiting
• loss of appetite
• changes in urine output
• fluid retention
• anemia (a decrease in red blood cells)

• decreased sex drive
• sudden rise in potassium levels (hyperkalemia)
• inflammation of the pericardium (fluid-filled sac that covers the heart)

What are the risk factors for developing kidney disease?
People with diabetes have a higher risk of developing kidney disease. Diabetes is the leading cause of kidney disease, accounting for about 44 percent of new cases. You may also be more likely to get kidney disease if you:
• have high blood pressure
• have other family members with chronic kidney disease
• are elderly
• are of African, Hispanic, Asian, or American Indian descent

How is kidney disease diagnosed?
Your doctor will first determine whether you belong in any of the high-risk groups. They will then run some tests to see if your kidneys are functioning properly. These tests may include:
Glomerular filtration rate (GFR)
This test will measure how well your kidneys are working and determine the stage of kidney disease.

Ultrasound or computed tomography (CT) Scan
Ultrasounds and CT scans produce clear images of your kidneys and urinary tract. The pictures allow your doctor to see if your kidneys are too small or large. They can also show any tumors or structural problems that may be present.

Kidney biopsy
During a kidney biopsy, your doctor will remove a small piece of tissue from your kidney while you're sedated. The tissue sample can help your doctor determine the type of kidney disease you have and how much damage has occurred.

Urine test
Your doctor may request a urine sample to test for albumin. Albumin is a protein that can be passed into your urine when your kidneys are damaged.

Blood creatinine test
Creatinine is a waste product. It's released into the blood when creatine (a molecule stored in muscle) is broken down. The levels of creatinine in your blood will increase if your kidneys aren't working properly.

How is kidney disease treated?
Treatment for kidney disease usually focuses on controlling the underlying cause of the disease.

This means your doctor will help you better manage your blood pressure, blood sugar, and cholesterol levels. They may use one or more of the following methods to treat kidney disease.

Drugs and medication

Your doctor will either prescribe angiotensin-converting enzyme (ACE) inhibitors, such as lisinopril and ramipril, or angiotensin receptor blockers (ARBs), such as irbesartan and olmesartan. These are blood pressure medications that can slow the progression of kidney disease. Your doctor may prescribe these medications to preserve kidney function, even if you don't have high blood pressure.

You may also be treated with cholesterol drugs (such as simvastatin). These medications can reduce blood cholesterol levels and help maintain kidney health. Depending on your symptoms, your doctor may also prescribe drugs to relieve swelling and treat anemia (decrease in the number of red blood cells).

Dietary and lifestyle changes

Making changes to your diet is just as important as taking medication. Adopting a healthy lifestyle can help prevent many of the underlying causes of kidney disease. Your doctor may recommend that you:

• control diabetes through insulin injections
• cut back on foods high in cholesterol

• cut back on salt
• start a heart-healthy diet that includes fresh fruits, veggies, whole grains, and low-fat dairy products
• limit alcohol consumption
• quit smoking
• increase physical activity
• lose weight

Dialysis and kidney disease
Dialysis is an artificial method of filtering the blood. It's used when someone's kidneys have failed or are close to failing. Many people with late-stage kidney disease must go on dialysis permanently or until a donor kidney is found.

There are two types of dialysis: hemodialysis and peritoneal dialysis.
Hemodialysis
In hemodialysis, the blood is pumped through a special machine that filters out waste products and fluid. Hemodialysis is done at your home or in a hospital or dialysis center. Most people have three sessions per week, with each session lasting three to five hours. However, hemodialysis can also be done in shorter, more frequent sessions.
Several weeks before starting hemodialysis, most people will have surgery to create an

arteriovenous (AV) fistula. An AV fistula is created by connecting an artery and a vein just below the skin, typically in the forearm. The larger blood vessel allows an increased amount of blood to flow continuously through the body during hemodialysis treatment. This means more blood can be filtered and purified. An arteriovenous graft (a looped, plastic tube) may be implanted and used for the same purpose if an artery and vein can't be joined together.

The most common side effects of hemodialysis are low blood pressure, muscle cramping, and itching.

Peritoneal dialysis

In peritoneal dialysis, the peritoneum (membrane that lines the abdominal wall) stands in for the kidneys. A tube is implanted and used to fill the abdomen with a fluid called dialysate. Waste products in the blood flow from the peritoneum into the dialysate. The dialysate is then drained from the abdomen.

There are two forms of peritoneal dialysis: continuous ambulatory peritonealdialysis, where the abdomen is filled and drained several times during the day, and continuous cycler-assisted peritoneal dialysis, which uses a machine to cycle the fluid in and out of the abdomen at night while the person sleeps.

The most common side effects of peritoneal dialysis are infections in the abdominal cavity or in the area where the tube was implanted. Other side effects may include weight gain and hernias. A hernia is when the intestine pushes through a weak spot or tear in the lower abdominal wall.

What is the long-term outlook for someone with kidney disease?
Kidney disease normally does not go away once it's diagnosed. The best way to maintain kidney health is to adopt a healthy lifestyle and follow your doctor's advice. Kidney disease can get worse over time. It may even lead to kidney failure. Kidney failure can be life-threatening if left untreated.

Kidney failure occurs when your kidneys are barely working or not working at all. This is managed by dialysis. Dialysis involves the use of a machine to filter waste from your blood. In some cases, your doctor may recommend a kidney transplant.

How can kidney disease be prevented?
Some risk factors for kidney disease — such as age, race, or family history — are impossible to control. However, there are measures you can take to help prevent kidney disease:

- drink plenty of water
- control blood sugar if you have diabetes
- control blood pressure
- reduce salt intake
- quit smoking

Be careful with over-the-counter drugs
You should always follow the dosage instructions for over-the-counter medications. Taking too much aspirin (Bayer) or ibuprofen (Advil, Motrin) can cause kidney damage. Call your doctor if the normal doses of these medications aren't controlling your pain effectively.

Get tested
Ask your doctor about getting a blood test for kidney problems. Kidney problems generally don't cause symptoms until they're more advanced. A basic metabolic panel (BMP) is a standard blood test that can be done as part of a routine medical exam. It checks your blood for creatinine or urea. These are chemicals that leak into the blood when the kidneys aren't working properly. A BMP can detect kidney problems early, when they're easier to treat. You should be tested annually if you have diabetes, heart disease, or high blood pressure.

Limit certain foods
Different chemicals in your food can contribute to certain types of kidney stones. These include:
• excessive sodium
• animal protein, such as beef and chicken
• citric acid, found in citrus fruits such as oranges, lemons, and grapefruits
• oxalate, a chemical found in beets, spinach, sweet potatoes, and chocolate

Ask about calcium
Talk to your doctor before taking a calcium supplement. Some calcium supplements have been linked to an increased risk of kidney stones.

Herbal Supplements and Kidney Disease
Is it safe to use herbal supplements if I have kidney disease?
You may think about using herbal supplements to help with any health concerns you may have, but as a patient with kidney disease, you should use caution with herbal supplements.
Use of herbal supplements is often unsafe if you have kidney disease since some herbal products can cause harm to your kidneys and even make your kidney disease worse. Also,

your kidneys cannot clear waste products that can build up in your body.

The herbal supplement market is a multi-million dollar business. You may hear from a friend or family member about an herbal supplement that they think has improved their health or well-being and they suggest it to you. While this advice may be fine for them, it can be dangerous for you with kidney disease.

What are the facts about herbal supplements?
The following facts about herbal supplements are true for everyone, with or without kidney disease. Herbal supplements often have more than one name: a common name and a plant name. Some common concerns include:

• The Food and Drug Administration (FDA) does not regulate herbal supplements for dose, content, or pureness.

• Some herbal supplements have aristolochic acid, which is harmful to kidneys.

• Herbal supplements made in other countries may have heavy metals.

• There are few studies to show if herbal supplements have real benefits and even less information in patients with kidney disease.

• Herbal supplements may interact with prescription medicines to either decrease or increase how the medicine works.

Which herbal supplements have potassium?
Potassium is a mineral that may need to be limited in the diet of people with kidney disease especially for those on dialysis. Herbal supplements that have potassium include:

Alfalfa American Ginseng Bai Zhi (root)

Bitter Melon (fruit, leaf) Black Mustard (leaf) Blessed Thistle

Chervit (leaf) Chicory (leaf) Chinese Boxthorn (leaf)

Coriander (leaf) Dandelion (root, leaf) Dulse

Evening Primrose Feverfew Garlic (leaf)

Genipap (fruit) Goto Kola Japanese Honeysuckle (flower)

Kelp Kudzu (shoot) Lemongrass

Mugwort Noni Papaya (leaf, fruit)

Purslane Sage (leaf) Safflower (flower) Sassafras

Scullcap Shepherd's Purse Stinging Nettle (leaf)

Turmeric (rhizome) Water Lotus

Which herbal supplements have phosphorus?
Phosphorus is a mineral that may need to be limited in the diet of people with kidney disease especially for those on dialysis. Some herbal supplements that have phosphorus include:

American Ginseng Bitter Melon Borage (leaf)

Buchu (leaf) Coriander (leaf) Evening Primrose

Feverfew Flaxseed (seed) Horseradish (root)

Indian Sorrel (seed) Milk Thistle Onion (leaf)
Pokeweed (shoot) Purslane Shepherd's Purse
Silk Cotton Tree (seed) Stinging Nettle (leaf)
Sunflower (seed)
Turmeric (rhizome) Water Lotus Yellow Dock

Which herbal supplements should I avoid if I have kidney disease?
Herbal supplements that are especially risky for patients with any stage of kidney disease, who are on dialysis or who have a kidney transplant include:
Astragalus Barberry Cat's Claw
Apium Graveolens Creatine Goldenrod
Horsetail Huperzinea Java Tea Leaf
Licorice Root Nettle, Stinging Nettle Oregon Grape Root
Parsley Root Pennyroyal Ruta Graveolens
Uva Ursi Yohimbe

What about herbal supplements that act like a "water pill"?
Some herbal supplements that act like a diuretic or "water pill" may cause "kidney irritation" or damage. These include bucha leaves and juniper berries. Uva Ursi and parsley capsules may also have bad side effects.

Can herbal supplements interfere with the other medicines I take?

Many herbal supplements can interact with prescription drugs. A few examples are St. Johns Wort, echinacea, ginkgo, garlic, ginseng, ginger, and blue cohosh. If you have a kidney transplant you are especially at risk, as any interaction between herbal supplements and medicines could put you at risk for losing your kidney.

Are there other health related issues for herbal supplements?

As with anyone, patients with kidney disease may have other health related issues. If you have a history of a bleeding disorder you are at high risk for bad reactions to herbal supplements. Women who are pregnant or lactating, as well as children, are also at high risk.

Best Foods for People with Kidney Disease

Kidney disease is a common problem affecting about 10% of the world's population.

The kidneys are small but powerful bean-shaped organs that perform many important functions.

They are responsible for filtering waste products, releasing hormones that regulate blood pressure, balancing fluids in the body, producing urine, and many other essential tasks.

There are various ways in which these vital organs can become damaged.

Diabetes and high blood pressure are the most common risk factors for kidney disease. However, obesity, smoking, genetics, gender, and age can also increase the risk.

Uncontrolled blood sugar and high blood pressure cause damage to blood vessels in the kidneys, reducing their ability to function optimally.

When the kidneys aren't working properly, waste builds up in the blood, including waste products from food.

Therefore, it's necessary for people with kidney disease to follow a special diet.

Diet and kidney disease

Dietary restrictions vary depending on the level of kidney damage.

For example, people in the early stages of kidney disease have different restrictions than those with kidney failure, also known as end-stage renal disease (ESRD).

If you have kidney disease, your health care provider will determine the best diet for your needs.

For most people with advanced kidney disease, it's important to follow a kidney-friendly diet that helps decrease the amount of waste in the blood.

This diet is often referred to as a renal diet.

It helps boost kidney function while preventing further damage.

While dietary restrictions vary, it's commonly recommended that all people with kidney disease restrict the following nutrients:

• Sodium. Sodium is found in many foods and a major component of table salt. Damaged kidneys can't filter out excess sodium, causing its blood levels to rise. It's often recommended to limit sodium to less than 2,000 mg per day.

• Potassium. Potassium plays many critical roles in the body, but those with kidney disease need to limit potassium to avoid dangerously high blood levels. It's usually recommended to limit potassium to less than 2,000 mg per day.

• Phosphorus. Damaged kidneys can't remove excess phosphorus, a mineral in many foods. High levels can cause damage to the body, so dietary phosphorus is restricted to less than 800–1,000 mg per day in most patients.

Protein is another nutrient that people with kidney disease may need to limit, as damaged kidneys can't clear out waste products from protein metabolism.

However, those with end-stage renal disease undergoing dialysis, a treatment that filters and cleans the blood, have greater protein needs.

Each person with kidney disease is different, which is why it's important to talk to your healthcare provider about your individual dietary needs.

Luckily, many delicious and healthy options are low in phosphorus, potassium, and sodium.

Here are 20 of the best foods for people with kidney disease.

1. Cauliflower

Cauliflower is a nutritious vegetable that's a good source of many nutrients, including vitamin C, vitamin K, and the B vitamin folate.

It's also full of anti-inflammatory compounds like indoles and is an excellent source of fiber.

Plus, mashed cauliflower can be used in place of potatoes for a low potassium side dish.

One cup (124 grams) of cooked cauliflower contains:

• sodium: 19 mg
• potassium: 176 mg
• phosphorus: 40 mg

2. Blueberries

Blueberries are packed with nutrients and one of the best sources of antioxidants you can eat.

In particular, these sweet berries contain antioxidants called anthocyanins, which may protect against heart disease, certain cancers, cognitive decline, and diabetes.

They also make a fantastic addition to a kidney-friendly diet, as they are low in sodium, phosphorus, and potassium.

One cup (148 grams) of fresh blueberries contains:

• sodium: 1.5 mg
• potassium: 114 mg
• phosphorus: 18 mg

3. Sea bass

Sea bass is a high ⬚uality protein that contains incredibly healthy fats called omega-3s.

Omega-3s help reduce inflammation and may help decrease the risk of cognitive decline, depression, and anxiety.

While all fish are high in phosphorus, sea bass contains lower amounts than other seafood.

However, it's important to consume small portions to keep your phosphorus levels in check.

Three ounces (85 grams) of cooked sea bass contain:

• sodium: 74 mg
• potassium: 279 mg
• phosphorus: 211 mg

4. Red grapes

Red grapes are not only delicious but also deliver a ton of nutrition in a small package.

They're high in vitamin C and contain antioxidants called flavonoids, which have been shown to reduce inflammation.

Additionally, red grapes are high in resveratrol, a type of flavonoid that has been shown to benefit heart health and protect against diabetes and cognitive decline.

These sweet fruits are kidney-friendly, with a half cup (75 grams) containing:

- sodium: 1.5 mg
- potassium: 144 mg
- phosphorus: 15 mg

5. Egg whites

Although egg yolks are very nutritious, they contain high amounts of phosphorus, making egg whites a better choice for people following a renal diet.

Egg whites provide a high quality, kidney-friendly source of protein.

Plus, they're an excellent choice for people undergoing dialysis treatment, who have higher protein needs but need to limit phosphorus.

Two large egg whites (66 grams) contain:

- sodium: 110 mg
- potassium: 108 mg
- phosphorus: 10 mg

6. Garlic

People with kidney problems are advised to limit the amount of sodium in their diet, including added salt.

Garlic provides a delicious alternative to salt, adding flavor to dishes while providing nutritional benefits.

It's a good source of manganese, vitamin C, and vitamin B6 and contains sulfur compounds that have anti-inflammatory properties.

Three cloves (9 grams) of garlic contain:

• sodium: 1.5 mg
• potassium: 36 mg
• phosphorus: 14 mg

7. Buckwheat

Many whole grains tend to be high in phosphorus, but buckwheat is a healthy exception.

Buckwheat is highly nutritious, providing a good amount of B vitamins, magnesium, iron, and fiber.

It's also a gluten-free grain, making buckwheat a good choice for people with celiac disease or gluten intolerance.

A half cup (84 grams) of cooked buckwheat contains:

• sodium: 3.5 mg
• potassium: 74 mg
• phosphorus: 59 mg

8. Olive oil

Olive oil is a healthy source of fat and phosphorus-free, making it a great option for people with kidney disease.

Frequently, people with advanced kidney disease have trouble keeping weight on, making healthy, high calorie foods like olive oil important.

The majority of fat in olive oil is a monounsaturated fat called oleic acid, which has anti-inflammatory properties.

What's more, monounsaturated fats are stable at high temperatures, making olive oil a healthy choice for cooking.

One tablespoon (13.5 grams) of olive oil contains:

- sodium: 0.3 mg
- potassium: 0.1 mg
- phosphorus: 0 mg

9. Bulgur

Bulgur is a whole grain wheat product that makes a terrific, kidney-friendly alternative to other whole grains that are high in phosphorus and potassium.

This nutritious grain is a good source of B vitamins, magnesium, iron, and manganese.

It's also an excellent source of plant-based protein and full of dietary fiber, which is important for digestive health.

A half-cup (91-gram) serving of bulgur contains:

- sodium: 4.5 mg
- potassium: 62 mg
- phosphorus: 36 mg

10. Cabbage

Cabbage belongs to the cruciferous vegetable family and is loaded with vitamins, minerals, and powerful plant compounds.

It's a great source of vitamin K, vitamin C, and many B vitamins.

Furthermore, it provides insoluble fiber, a type of fiber that keeps your digestive system healthy by promoting regular bowel movements and adding bulk to stool.

Plus, it's low in potassium, phosphorus, and sodium, with one cup (70 grams) of shredded cabbage containing:

- sodium: 13 mg
- potassium: 119 mg
- phosphorus: 18 mg

11. Skinless chicken

Although a limited protein intake is necessary for some people with kidney issues, providing the body with an adequate amount of high quality protein is vital for health.

Skinless chicken breast contains less phosphorus, potassium, and sodium than skin-on chicken.

When shopping for chicken, choose fresh chicken and avoid pre-made roasted chicken, as it contains large amounts of sodium and phosphorus.

Three ounces (84 grams) of skinless chicken breast contains:

• sodium: 63 mg
• potassium: 216 mg
• phosphorus: 192 mg

12. Bell peppers

Bell peppers contain an impressive amount of nutrients but are low in potassium, unlike many other vegetables.

These brightly colored peppers are loaded with the powerful antioxidant vitamin C.

In fact, one small red bell pepper (74 grams) contains 105% of the recommended intake of vitamin C.

They are also loaded with vitamin A, an important nutrient for immune function, which is often compromised in people with kidney disease.

One small red pepper (74 grams) contains:

• sodium: 3 mg
• potassium: 156 mg
• phosphorus: 19 mg

13. Onions

Onions are excellent for providing sodium-free flavor to renal-diet dishes.

Reducing salt intake can be challenging, making finding flavorful salt alternatives a must.

Sautéing onions with garlic and olive oil adds flavor to dishes without compromising your kidney health.

What's more, onions are high in vitamin C, manganese, and B vitamins and contain prebiotic fibers that help keep your digestive system healthy by feeding beneficial gut bacteria.

One small onion (70 grams) contains:
• sodium: 3 mg
• potassium: 102 mg
• phosphorus: 20 mg

14. Arugula

Many healthy greens like spinach and kale are high in potassium and difficult to fit into a renal diet.

However, arugula is a nutrient-dense green that is low in potassium, making it a good choice for kidney-friendly salads and side dishes.

Arugula is a good source of vitamin K and the minerals manganese and calcium, all of which are important for bone health.

This nutritious green also contains nitrates, which have been shown to lower blood pressure, an important benefit for those with kidney disease.

One cup (20 grams) of raw arugula contains:

- sodium: 6 mg
- potassium: 74 mg
- phosphorus: 10 mg

15. Macadamia nuts

Most nuts are high in phosphorus and not recommended for those following a renal diet.

However, macadamia nuts are a delicious option for people with kidney problems. They are much lower in phosphorus than popular nuts like peanuts and almonds.

They are also packed with healthy fats, B vitamins, magnesium, copper, iron, and manganese.

One ounce (28 grams) of macadamia nuts contains:

- sodium: 1.4 mg
- potassium: 103 mg
- phosphorus: 53 mg

16. Radish

Radishes are crunchy vegetables that make a healthy addition to a renal diet.

This is because they are very low in potassium and phosphorus but high in many other important nutrients.

Radishes are a great source of vitamin C, an antioxidant that has been shown to decrease the risk of heart disease and cataracts.

Additionally, their peppery taste makes a flavorful addition to low sodium dishes.

A half cup (58 grams) of sliced radishes contains:

• sodium: 23 mg
• potassium: 135 mg
• phosphorus: 12 mg

17. Turnips

Turnips are kidney-friendly and make an excellent replacement for vegetables that are higher in potassium like potatoes and winter squash.

These root vegetables are loaded with fiber and vitamin C. They are also a decent source of vitamin B6 and manganese.

They can be roasted or boiled and mashed for a healthy side dish that works well for a renal diet.

A half cup (78 grams) of cooked turnips contains:

• sodium: 12.5 mg
• potassium: 138 mg
• phosphorus: 20 mg

18. Pineapple

Many tropical fruits like oranges, bananas, and kiwis are very high in potassium.

Fortunately, pineapple makes a sweet, low potassium alternative for those with kidneys problems.

Plus, pineapple is rich in fiber, manganese, vitamin C, and bromelain, an enzyme that helps reduce inflammation.

One cup (165 grams) of pineapple chunks contains:

• sodium: 2 mg
• potassium: 180 mg
• phosphorus: 13 mg

19. Cranberries

Cranberries benefit both the urinary tract and kidneys.

These tiny, tart fruits contain phytonutrients called A-type proanthocyanidins, which prevent bacteria from sticking to the lining of the urinary tract and bladder, thus preventing infection.

This is helpful for those with kidney disease, as they have an increased risk of urinary tract infections.

Cranberries can be eaten dried, cooked, fresh, or as a juice. They are very low in potassium, phosphorus, and sodium.

One cup (100 grams) of fresh cranberries contains:

- sodium: 2 mg
- potassium: 80 mg
- phosphorus: 11 mg

20. Shiitake mushrooms

Shiitake mushrooms are a savory ingredient that can be used as a plant-based meat substitute for those on a renal diet who need to limit protein.

They are an excellent source of B vitamins, copper, manganese, and selenium.

In addition, they provide a good amount of plant-based protein and dietary fiber.

Shiitake mushrooms are lower in potassium than portobello and white button mushrooms, making them a smart choice for those following a renal diet.

One cup (145 grams) of cooked shiitake mushroom contains:

- sodium: 6 mg
- potassium: 170 mg
- phosphorus: 42 mg

Other Herbs For Kidneys

Here are 10 herbs and natural remedies that have been studied and are believed to be beneficial for the kidneys:

10 Herbs For Kidneys

Green Tea

The young, "unfermented" leaves of the tea plant (Camellia sinensis) are widely considered to have great nutritional ualities. Most green teas are unfermented or very lightly fermented, as opposed to oolong teas which are semi-fermented and black teas which are fully fermented.

Tea has been shown to possess anti-inflammatory, astringent and diuretic properties. It also contains compounds called polyphenols that have been known to inhibit kidney stones and even prevent certain cancers. [2] It is these polyphenols that are widely investigated for their anti-oxidant activities to prevent diseases caused by oxidative stress like kidney related disorders. As one recent Japanese study has shown, the biological activities and low toxicity of polyphenols have beneficial effects on pathological states related to oxidative stress renal disease.

Couch Grass

Rich in polysaccharides, volatile oils, mucilages and other nutrients, couch grass has been traditionally used to increase urine production and treat urinary tract infections like cystitis and urethritis. It has diuretic, demulcent and antibacterial properties, couch grass is therefore also used to partially dissolve kidney stones. Consequently, researchers in Italy discovered that when combined with potassium citrate, the dry extract of couch grass significantly reduced the total number and size of urinary stones among the treated group after a 5 month follow up period in a randomized controlled study.

Rehmannia

Rehmannia is an herb that is less well known in the West but has been used in Traditional Chinese Medicine since ancient times. The steamed roots of rehmannia have been widely used to fight various renal diseases. A 2009 study revealed that this herb has reno-protective effects on progressive renal failure by reducing angiotensin II, AT1 receptor, and by regulating TGF-β1 and type IV collagen expression. Phytosterols, antioxidants, along with iridoid glycosides are reported to be responsible for rehmannia's therapeutic benefits on the kidneys.

Banaba

An ornamental plant indigenous to Australia, India and tropical countries in Southeast Asia, banaba has been used since ancient times as a natural diuretic and as a remedy for kidney and bladder problems. While much research is focused on the herb's high levels of corosolic acid and how this may improve blood sugar levels among type II diabetics, the leaves of banaba have also been used to relieve urinary tract infections. Evidence also suggests regular intake of banaba leaf tea can alleviate the discomfort associated with kidney stones and help prevent gallbladder stones.

Java Tea (Orthosiphon stamineus)
Listed in French, Indonesian, Dutch and Swiss pharmacopoeias as a remedy for kidney ailments, java teahas diuretic properties and increases the kidney's ability to eliminate nitrogen-containing compounds. Some experts believe java tea is an effective treatment against kidney stones, kidney infections and for promoting renal functions because of the flavones, glycoside, volatile oil and potassium it contains. Recent studies have also revealed that java tea's caffeic acid and rosmarinic content can trigger helpful biological mechanisms. Java tea is also thought to treat gout, diabetes and rheumatism.

Cranberries
Initially thought only to be beneficial for treating urinary tract infections, recent scientific studies revealed that cranberries may

also contribute to preventing the formation of kidney stones. Research shows that cranberries are good sources of quinic acid, a very acidic substance which the body cannot dissolve. This substance helps make urine more acidic thereby preventing the phosphate and calcium ions from forming kidney stones.

Dandelion

When made into tea, dandelion can be a helpful assistant to the liver and the kidneys. In addition to its diuretic properties, dandelion is an excellent source of nutrients such as zinc, potassium, iron, andVitamins A, C, D and B-Complex. The roots of dandelion contain active ingredients that are thought may help dissolve kidney stones.

Ginger

For more than 2,000 years, ginger has been used to treat different types of ailments including renal disorders. Scientific experimental evidence suggests that ginger contains active constituents that activate antioxidant pathways resulting to increased renal protection.

As a good reservoir of valuable dietary elements like Vitamin C, folic acid, Vitamin B3, iron, calcium and protein, ginger is a wonderful

herb that also helps dissolve kidney stones.
stones.

Cucumber
Cucumber is a vegetable consist of 97% water.
When made into juice or eaten raw, cucumbers
are excellent sources of valuable nutrients like
Vitamin A, Vitamin C, lutein, beta carotene,
calcium, magnesium, protein, phosphorus and
calcium.
Noted for their diuretic and laxative properties,
cucumber is highly recommended to people
suffering from kidney problems. This vegetable
helps to eliminate harmful toxins in the kidneys
as well as dissolve bladder and kidney stones.
Onion
Research shows that onions can be helpful in
eliminating pain associated with kidney stones.
Regular intake of onion juice is thought to be
useful for making kidney stones pass within at
least 24 hours.

Kidney Cleansing Herbs : Benefits, Best Uses &
Risks
Many kidney health supplements contain
kidney cleansing herbs claimed to cleanse,
detox and flush the kidneys. Some of the herbs
for kidneys can be very effective to detox the
kidneys and the urinary tract. Many herbs,

however, have very little evidence on their safety or effectiveness. In some cases, they can even cause side effects and kidney detox symptoms.

In this review, we share the best most commonly used herbs for kidneys, that are shown to be both safe and effective. We cover their main benefits and recommended use. We hope this guide will help your journey to a safe, effective and happy cleanse.

Chanca Piedra
Main benefits: dissolves kidney stones.
We start the list of the kidney cleansing herbs with the most famous herb for kidney health: Chanca piedra (Phyllanthus niruri).

Also known as stonebreaker, Chanca piedra has a long history of traditional use for kidney, liver and gallbladder health. A growing number of evidence suggests that Chanca piedra has the ability to dissolve kidney stones. (Hence the name).

According to the research data:
Chanca piedra was shown to interfere with many stages of kidney stone formation, reduce the stone crystals aggregation and modify the kidney stone structure and composition.

Recommendation: Chanca piedra has long traditional use for kidney and liver health. This use is also supported by published studies. If you consider to add kidney cleansing herbs as a part of your kidney cleanse, Chanca piedra would be our first pick.

Horsetail
Main benefits: diuretic, increases urine flow.
Second on the list and another kidney cleanse herb we like to include in the kidney cleanse, is Horsetail (E?uisetum arvense).
The long traditional use and research data all suggest that Horsetail has a very powerful yet safe diuretic effect. So it can safely increase the urine flow which helps to flush, cleanse and detox the kidneys, with no negative effect on the kidneys, liver, or the urinary excretion of electrolytes and catabolites [3].
Recommendation: Horsetail offers a safe and effective way to increase urine flow during the kidney cleanse, which can enhance the effects other kidney cleansing herbs. For this reason, it is often combined with Chanca piedra.

Hydrangea Root
Main benefits: overall kidney & urinary tract health.
Another potent kidney cleansing herb that also has solid evidence on its safety and effectiveness is hydrangea root.

The old cherokee native americans and later the settlers, used a decoction of hydrangea for kidney stones with great success. In his book, advanced course in herbology, Dr. Edward Shook stated that:

Hydrangea herb is a powerful solvent of stone and calculous deposits, not only in the renal organs, but in every part of the organism, wherever they may be located. Therefore it is destined to become a universal remedy for phosphaturia, cystitis, alkaline urine, stony deposits, deposits of oxalate of calcium and others.

These benefits of Hydrangea for kidney health are further supported by the medical community. Hydrangea showed anti-inflammation and antioxidation effects and was able to improve and protect the kidneys function..

Recommendation: Hydrangea herb offers an effective and safe way that can enhance the entire kidney and urinary tract. If you consider taking herbs for kidney health, we highly recommend to look for Hydrangea as well.

Uva Ursi
Main benefits: prevents urinary tract infections (UTIs).

Another kidney cleansing herbs superstar we recommend to include in the kidney cleanse is Uva ursi. Also known as arctostaphylos, bearberry, and bear's grape, this herb has a long history of medicinal use for cleansing the kidneys and the urinary tract.

What about the science? The leaf extract of uva ursi has been approved for use for urinary tract inflammation by the German Federal Institute for Drugs. The research data suggests that uva ursi has natural diuretic, urinary antiseptic, astringent and anti-inflammatory properties.
Recommendation: Uva ursi may help as a natural way to prevent urinary tract infections (UTI). For this reason, we like to include Uva ursi in the kidney cleanse together with other kidney cleansing herbs, as an extra support for the urinary system function.

Marshmallow Root
Main benefits: increases urine secretion & soothes urinary tract.
Marshmallow root (Althaea officinalis) is well known for its natural diuretic properties, along with an ability to relieve internal irritation and inflammation in the urinary tract.
These two benefits, make marshmallow root an excellent fit for the kidney cleanse; it can help

to flush the kidneys on one hand, while also relieves and soothes inflammation in the urinary tract.

Recommendation: Marshmallow root offers a safe and effective way to promote kidney and urinary tract health. Based on our experience, using Marshmallow root can enhance the effects other kidney cleansing herbs.

Dandelion

Main benefits: diuretic.

One famous kidney cleanse herb you can actually get fresh at the stores is Dandelion (Taraxacum officinale).

Due to its potent natural diuretic properties and high availability, you can find dandelion in many kidney cleanse products. Both in supplements and tea forms.

The historical evidence of using dandelion as a natural diuretic takes us over 2000 years back, seen in both traditional chinese and ayurvedic medicine. Human studies also support the benefits of dandelion for kidney health. As research data suggests, consuming a fresh leaf extract of dandelion increases the freuency of urination.

We like to use dandelions in kidney cleanse recipes, especially teas. A good example is our Dandelion Turmeric Lemon Kidney Cleanse Tea.

Recommendation: Dandelion may offer a natural and safe way to enhance the elimination of excess fluids by the kidneys. If you can get it fresh, you may want to try to make a kidney cleanse tea at home.

Natural Kidney Cleanse Protocol
The idea of the kidney cleanse is simple: you start your day with a liquid diet: kidney cleanse drink for breakfast, and juice for lunch. You have a kidney cleanse smoothie for the afternoon and eat a kidney cleansing meal for dinner.

Chapter 14: Treatment And Prevention

Kidney conditions are ⬚uiet killers. They might cause modern loss of kidney function resulting in kidney failure and also inevitably demand dialysis or kidney transplant to suffer life. Since of the high expense and also potential problems of absence of availability in establishing countries, only 5 -10% of patients with kidney failure are privileged ade⬚uate to obtain clear-cut therapy choices such as dialysis and also kidney hair transplant, while the rest pass away without getting any conclusive treatment. Chronic kidney disease (CKD) is extremely typical and also has no remedy, so avoidance is the only choice. Early discovery and therapy can usually maintain CKD from worsening, and also can protect against or postpone the re⬚uirement for definitive therapy.

Kidney Failure And Its Treatment

Kidney failure additionally called renal failure. It is a critical disease which can have a primary impact on life, and also can become dangerous. However, it can be cured.

Kidney failure is additionally related to a rise in the amount of water in the body, which can impact the swelling of the cells. Healthy and balanced kidneys wash your blood by removing excess fluid, minerals, and wastes. They make hormonal agents that safeguard your bones strong as well as your blood well also. If the organs are damaged, they don't run properly.

This is called kidney failure. It is a state in which the kidneys fail to function completely.

Kidney failure can generally be divided into 2 kinds: severe kidney failing as well as persistent kidney disease. Acute failure is the hasty loss of the capacity of the kidneys to remove waste as well as intentional urine without shedding electrolytes.

The kind of kidney failing (persistent vs. acute) is developed by the trend in the serum creatinine. Various other things that potentially will help to distinguish intensely and also persistent kidney disease include the visibility of anemia and also the kidney dimension on ultrasound. Enduring, i.e. chronic, kidney disease, commonly causes anemia and little kidney size.

At least, there are three choices when treating kidney failure:

1. Hemodialysis
2. Peritoneal dialysis
3. Kidney transplant

Every therapy has advantages as well as disadvantages. Regardless of which treatment you select, you'll have to make some modifications in your life, consisting of how you eat and also prepare your activities. Yet with the help of a doctor, family members, and good friends, the majority people with kidney failure can run completely satisfied as well as energetic lives.

For a suitable individual at the ideal time, a transplant is the finest treatment for kidney failure. If it operates effectively the person will be total without dialysis. Many people with kidney failure are proper for a transplant.

Kidney failure can happen quickly (days) or more unhurriedly (months or years). A lot of conditions can produce kidneys to fail, making up diabetes and high blood pressure. Lots of individuals with chronic kidney failing necessitate take medications, and also lots of demand dialysis.

Kidney Failure Treatment Without Dialysis

Kidney failing might set in as a result of several possible reasons consisting of long term use of over-the-counter and also prescription medications, health problems, exposure to chemicals over an extended period of time. Symptoms of kidney failure include vomiting, queasiness, persistent back troubles, and blood or protein in pee. Individuals can go with expensive choices like transplant or dialysis or for kidney failure therapy without dialysis

Techniques of kidney failing treatment without dialysis.

Right here are a couple of ways of dealing with kidney failure without choosing dialysis or transplant:

Consist of such food products in your diet plan that can be absorbed easily by the body. Stay clear of foodstuff, which puts tension on the kidneys for obtaining digested.

Specific natural herbs aid in detoxification of kidneys and boost their health and wellness. Before beginning usage of any one of over such herbs, do not fail to remember consulting your medical professional, particularly if you are taking prescription medicines.

Hoelen is one more herb that can confirm to be useful for kidney clients. Three to six grams of the dried out herb will certainly be excellent sufficient for preventing buildup of lesions in the kidney.

Cranberries: Urinary tract infections can be protected against by eating cranberry juice. Pure, bitter cranberry juice ought to be picked instead of cranberry juice mixed drink as the latter has high sugar levels.

4. Flaxseed: A whole lot has actually been claimed and blogged about exactly how efficiently flaxseed sustains kidney functions. In fact, flaxseed is abundant in omega-3 fatty acids as well as alpha-linolenic acid, which offers

enough ꞯuantity of assistance to the kidneys. These 2 substances are fairly efficient in stopping inflammation and obstructing of arteries.

Marshmallow: Kidney individuals should seriously consider consuming alcohol marshmallows for increasing kidney features. Drinking one quart of marshmallow daily is rather efficient in cleaning the kidneys. This techniꞯue can benefit people of kidney stones.

Kidney failure people need to prevent specific food products. Such food things consist of those with high salt web content. Oregano, basil, or parsley can be made use of to substitute salt for flavoring the food. Salad dressings, canned foods, barbeꞯue sauce, bacon and also various other food items having high salt web content must be avoided.

As shown by the above lines, one can conꞯuer kidney failure with specific easy remedies. Kidney failing treatment without dialysis is ꞯuite feasible. All you reꞯuire is some expertise and also lots of specialist suggestions.

How To Prevent Kidney Failure

For those who experience kidney disease, you will certainly understand just how essential it is to protect against kidney failing Kidney condition can be both long-term and also short-lived. This can be called severe kidney failure/acute renal failure or persistent kidney failure.

The difference between acute as well as chronic renal failure.

With acute kidney failure, the function of the kidneys is swiftly lost and can happen from numerous anxieties on the body, a lot of which are associated with diet plan. Others are indirectly associated with diet, being brought on by another condition or ailment. There are several categories of intense kidney disease as well as is popularized into the complying with groups:

Usual Pre-renal Causes of Kidney Disease

• dehydration from excess liquid loss (diarrhea, influenza, gastroenteritis, sweating).

• dehydration from the absence of fluid intake.

• hypovolemia from excess blood loss.

• obstruction of kidney arteries, as well as veins, are creating irregular blood circulation.

• pain reliever, various other medication as well as excess sodium/potassium/protein.

Usual Post-renal Causes of Renal Failure.

• Having any type of constraint in the bladder can create back-flow to the kidneys. This can create a collection of occasions, from infection to totally damaging the kidneys due to the excess pressure.

- Blockages, cysts, tumors in the abdominal area can create obstructions around the ureters.
- Other age-relevant obstructions, consisting of cancers and also other tumors around the bladder.
- Having kidney rocks does not directly influence kidney failure but does boost the risk; however, having a great deal of added strain on the kidneys.

Typical Causes of Kidney Damage.

- Toxic Medications are discovered in specific prescription antibiotics, ibuprofen, some anti-inflammatory medicines, iodine and also radiology medications.
- Sepsis can happen if the body's body immune system is fighting infection. This can create the kidneys to close down because of this.
- Muscle malfunction can cause muscle mass fibers, which are damaged to clog filtration of the kidneys. This can generally get on established by serious injury as well as burns to the body.
- inflammation of the kidney filtering system - the glomeruli.

Typical Causes of Chronic Kidney Failure.

Many problems noted above can cause chronic kidney failure.

- continuous hypertension.
- people are suffering diabetes.
- persistent glomerulonephritis.
- kidney stones.
- prostate disease or prostate cancer.
- reflux nephropathy.
- polycystic problems.

HOW TO CURE KIDNEY DISEASE NATURALLY

If you've been diagnosed with Chronic Kidney Disease lately, you probably have a lot of unanswered concerns in your mind. In the list of "ifs, buts, what're whys and just how's" one of the most vital inquiries you re?uire to deal with is - What next?

Kidney disease treatments include prescription drugs, dialysis as well as transplant. All the treatment measures stated are pharmaceutical approaches and also not natural condition therapies.

There is a lot of individuals on the planet today that experience from kidney condition as well as numerous really feel that there is no expect recuperation or even a somewhat regular lifestyle. This might have been real a few years earlier, but today there are people available searching for different techni🔲ues and useful suggestions for dealing with all different kinds of kidney diseases.

This section loses light on all-natural therapies for renal issues.

Kidney disease natural treatments include nutritional changes, usage of the natural herb, and also important oils.

1 Diet:

Diet regimen is a vital component of chronic kidney disease therapy. A lot of dietitians advise preventing foods abundant in salt. This includes salty snacks like crackers, tinned vegetables, as well as canned soups, processed cheeses, as well as meats and icy dinners. Eat lower potassium foods. Fruits such as apples, grapes, watermelons, and also strawberries and vegetables such as cabbages and environment-friendly beans are instances of reduced potassium foods. You need to stay clear of foods such as bananas, tomatoes, oranges, potatoes as well as spinach. Protein is re🔲uired for muscle growth and also toughness. However, it is not a valuable option for renal troubles. A dietician will certainly make referrals of the maximum 🔲uantity of grams of proteins you ought to eat daily.

2 Home Remedies:

Apple Cider Vinegar, Baking soft drink, and corn silk are natural substances to recover kidney infections. A pinch of cooking soft drink contributed to a glass of water restores the acid-base eॹuilibrium of pee. You need to drink bitter cranberry juice every day. It prevents the facility of germs by making the pee acidic. Juniper berries achieve the very same impact. An additional all-natural remedy is to eat one husk of garlic every day. Utilize a home heating pad to eliminate discomfort triggered by kidney conditions.

3 Herbal Treatments:

A variety of natural herbs, a lot of obtained from Chinese herbal remedies, have actually aided solve or at least offer remedy for kidney issues. Numerous amongst these are back by scientific researches. Herbs operate in different ways. Some are anti-inflammatory and also anti-bacterial representatives, while certain herbs help the kidneys eliminate waste products. Kidney advantageous herbs are Dandelion root and also Lei Gong Teng. Organic therapies reॹuire details precautions. One needs to take them in the dose and also kindly suggested by a professional of natural medicine. You need likewise to keep the nephrologist managing your case informed on making use of such natural treatments.

4 Preventive Measures

Avoidance is constantly much better than treatment. Follow these ideas to avoid the start of a kidney condition or infection.

- You can drink alcohol, however, in moderation.

- Over-the-counter and also prescription drugs are made use of to dealt with health and wellness conditions. Long term usage starts kidney damage. Drugs need to be absorbed the prescribed way just.

- Quit cigarette smoking. It is the most effective health choice you can make, not only for your kidneys yet likewise for your lungs.

- Obesity, like diabetes and hypertension, increases health complications. Keep healthy and balanced weight by consuming right and also exercising regularly.

Kidney conditions need not be taken gently. A very early medical diagnosis and suitable kidney disease therapy measures will boost feature and increase the top ⬚uality of your life.

Calcium And Kidney Stones - How To Pass Kidney Stones Naturally

Calcium, as well as kidney rocks, go with each other. Actually, about 9 in every 10 kidney stones are made up of calcium. This is fantastic information because calcium kidney rocks are the most basic to treat normally as well as they can actually be dissolved.

In this section, you will certainly learn exactly how to pass them normally with straightforward treatments and common foods.

Consume Plenty of Water for Kidney Stones

I am guessing that you have already tried consuming a lot of water for treating you your condition. You ought to ⬚uickly begin doing this if you have not. Water is very important for the kidneys to operate effectively.

Actually, many calcium rocks are the result of not consuming alcohol sufficient water to purge the calcium (called dehydration). But besides drinking a lot of water, there are likewise other things that you can do today.

Pass Calcium Kidney Stones Naturally

1. Consume a minimum of 100 ounces of water the whole day. You should drink at the very least 1 mug for each hour you are awake.

2. Consuming lemon day-to-day (include in water) can also benefit the kidneys by assisting the rocks dissolve. The citric acid (in lemons) can be valuable for dissolving calcium deposits in the kidneys.

3. Exercise daily to change the stones and also assist them to pass.

4. Eating a lot of fruits, veggies, entire grains, and bran can give fiber also to assist purge the kidneys. You need to eat at least 7 servings of fruits or veggies daily.

5. Resting at the very least 8 hours an evening will also aid.

6. Some studies show that taking a magnesium supplement at 300 to 350 mg daily can additionally be advantageous.

7. You should additionally avoid eating a lot of sugar, which has been linked with a higher threat of this disease.

8. Phosphoric acid is, without a doubt the greatest dissolvent for passing calcium rocks. Learn what beverages have this crucial acid.

HOW TO AVOID DIALYSIS THROUGH DRUG TREATMENTS

It's terrifying to be diagnosed with persistent kidney disease (CKD) if you find out in the very early stages of the disease, there are actions you can take to prolong kidney feature. Opportunities are great; you can still appreciate a healthful top quality of life with kidney condition if you function closely with your medical professional.

Following health techniques, remaining on the work as well as remaining to take pleasure in social tasks are methods a person can feel in control of their condition. Along with doing everything physically and clinically possible to extend kidney features, having a job with wellness insurance policy provides security that income, as well as wellness advantages, will certainly be offered.

Dialysis

Dialysis is a therapy for kidney failure. There are two sorts of dialysis: hemodialysis as well as peritoneal dialysis. Hemodialysis makes use of a machine to cleanse your blood. This sort of dialysis can be done at a dialysis center or in a tidy area in your home. Hemodialysis that is performed in a dialysis center is called in-center hemodialysis, as well as it is one of the most common treatments for kidney failure. Peritoneal dialysis uses the lining of your abdomen (stubborn belly area), called your abdominal muscle, as a filter to clean your blood. This sort of dialysis can be done anywhere that is completely dry and also tidy.

Dialysis utilizes devices to clean your blood as well as do a few of the jobs (around 10%) that healthy and balanced kidneys do. Dialysis can aid with signs brought on by kidney failure; however if you have various other medical conditions, e.g. stroke, Parkinson's disease, peripheral vascular condition, frailty, or dementia, dialysis will not assist with the signs and symptoms that they create, as well as might also make them worse. Dialysis does not stop your kidney function wearing away better; as a matter of fact, it can often make it worsen quicker.

Dialysis can be a troublesome treatment and might minimize high quality of life, specifically in patients with various other medical conditions. Dialysis therapy does not constantly prolong life in people with other clinical conditions; even if it does, a lot of the additional days of life obtained might be spent in health center.

After taking these and also other variables into consideration, some people pick not to begin dialysis; however instead select energetic encouraging treatment (in some cases referred to as traditional, optimal traditional or responsive care).

There are many reasons for CKD; there are certain referrals that, when complied with, can aid a person in delay kidney failure, which leads to dialysis or kidney transplant.

The two primary reasons for CKD in Americans are diabetes and high blood pressure. This disease should be controlled-- or prevented-- to assist extend kidney function

Diabetes and also extending kidney feature

Diabetics require to maintain their blood sugar level in an acceptable variety as well as take all physician-prescribed medicines. Furthermore, the hemoglobin A1c must be maintained listed below 6.5 percent, and also kidney function tests need to be done at the very least yearly. Studies have shown that specific hypertension medications can protect the kidneys of individuals with diabetic issues, also if they have typical high blood pressure.

High blood pressure and prolonging kidney features.

Individuals with hypertension, also understood as hypertension, should take their blood stress medication as directed by their physician. The National Heart, Lung, and also Blood Institute recommends that blood pressure remains in control at 125/75 or lower for those with kidney troubles, which are not diabetic persons, or 130/85 or lower for those with diabetes.

Various other disease that causes kidney damage

Various other disease that can damage kidneys includes IgA nephropathy, lupus as well as glomerulonephritis. With these diseases the body's immune system overacts, and also inflammation happens in the kidneys. To reduce the disease process, a medical professional might recommend steroids and other drugs.

CKD might likewise be prompted by infections, obstructions, and medications that damage the kidneys. Infections can often be cleared up with antibiotics. Obstructions might be eliminated with surgical procedures or other treatments. Particular medicines, such as prescription and also non-prescription painkillers, some anti-biotics as well as comparison dye (utilized in medical screening) may have negative effects on the kidneys. A client needs to talk their physicians that they have CKD and also supply a checklist of all the medications they are taking, consisting of over-the-counter drugs, to stop further kidney damage.

Actions to prolong kidney function

No matter exactly how an individual creates CKD, there are actions an individual can take to extend kidney features. Cigarette smoking creates uicker progression of kidney condition. As a result, it's advised that those with kidney disease stop smoking. Lots of doctors believe that also avoiding much protein as well as phosphorus in the diet might additionally slow the development of kidney disease.

Remember, your kidney problem is special. You can speak with your medical professional and work with your wellness treatment group for personalized tips on how to extend your kidney function. A constant and also open dialog will certainly create the most effective results. As discussing your medical condition, talk to your medical professional about your sensations as well as ask for suggestions on exactly how to speak with your household about CKD. Your health care group wishes to assist keep you healthy both literally and also psychologically.

How to delay the onset of dialysis-- at a glance

- Eat right as well as lose excess weight
- Exercise regularly
- Don't smoke
- Avoid excess salt in your diet
- Control of hypertension
- Control diabetes mellitus
- Stay on the job as well as keep your medical insurance
- Talk with your healthcare team

NUTRITION GUIDE FOR KIDNEY PATIENTS

If you have persistent kidney disease (CKD), it's important to see what you consume. Due to the fact that your kidneys can't get rid of waste items from your body like they should, that's. A kidney-friendly diet regimen can assist you to stay much healthier, much longer.

What's a Kidney-Friendly Diet?

It's a means of consuming that aids shield your kidneys from more damages. It suggests restricting some foods as well as liquids, so certain minerals do not develop in your body. At the very same time, you'll need to make certain you obtain the ideal equilibrium of protein, minerals, calories, and also vitamins.

If you're at the beginning of CKD, there may be few, if any type of, limits on what you can consume. But as your disease becomes worse, you'll need to be more careful regarding what you place into your body.

Your medical professional may suggest you collaborate with a dietitian to pick foods that are easy on your kidneys.

Eating correctly is essential for kidney health and wellness. Individuals with kidney disease need to keep an eye on the consumption of phosphorus, potassium, and sodium, especially.

Individuals with kidney disease might need to control a number of essential nutrients. The complying with info will aid you in adjusting your diet plan.

Please review your particular and individual diet plan reuires with your doctor or dietitian.

Right here are some points he may recommend:

Salt

Sodium is a mineral discovered in salt (salt chloride), and also it is widely utilized in cooking. Salt is just one of the most commonly utilized spices, and it requires time to get made use of to lowering the salt in your diet. Nevertheless, reducing salt/sodium is a crucial device in regulating your kidney disease.

- Do not use salt when cooking food.

- Do not place salt on food when you consume.

- Learn to read food tags. Stay clear of foods that have greater than 300mg salt per serving (or 600mg for a full frozen supper). Stay clear of foods that have salt in the very first 4 or 5 products in the component listing.

- Do not consume pork, bacon, sausage, hot canines, luncheon meat, hen tenders or nuggets, or routine tinned soup. Just consume soups that have labels stating the sodium level is lowered-- and also just consume 1 mug-- not kinds.

Conclusion

Thank you again for purchasing this book!
I hope this book was able to help you to get rid of your kidney stones and prevent them from coming back in the future.
The next step is to DRINK WATER.
With several ways to get rid of a kidney stone; there will be at least one simple and safe approach that levels to the passion of the individual. One way is the daily need and non-controversial action of the sufferer to drink enough water, especially when exposed to environment that is prone to dehydration.
While you are sweating profusely, the liquid of the body becomes more concentrated including the urine. This is a danger for stones to precipitate in your kidney.
DRINK enough water, NOT soda, as it will cause kidney stones as your urine turns to pale yellow. The daily intake of water varies depending on your fluid requirements. By simply maintaining light- colored urine, you are on your way toward preventing kidney stones.
Although, there are a number of medical procedures and surgical techniques to treat kidney stones; however, physicians typically avoid the procedure unless there is no other choice. This is an advantage as American

patients had been facing several problems due to medical errors.

You are the master of your fate if you prefer the natural way of passing kidney stone or to deal with this often very painful problem in the first place.

Opt for the best and most natural ways to prevent kidney stones that do not involve pain, money and changing your lifestyle:

Maintain a diet based on the unique nutritional requirement of your body, avoid prescription drugs that offer false promises of joy and keep away from soy and sugar.

Thank you and good luck!

www.ingramcontent.com/pod-product-compliance
Lightning Source LLC
Chambersburg PA
CBHW060330030426
42336CB00011B/1271